MAKING SENSE OF LUNG FUNCTION TESTS

A HANDS-ON GUIDE

Jonathan H Dakin
BSc MRCP
Consultant Respiratory Physician,
Queen Alexandra Hospital, Portsmouth, UK

Elena N Kourteli
FRCA
Consultant Anaesthetist, St George's Hospital, London, UK

and

Robert J D Winter
MD FRCP
Consultant Respiratory Physician,
Addenbrooke's Hospital and Papworth Hospital, Cambridge, UK

A member of the Hodder Headline Group
LONDON

First published in Great Britain in 2003 by
Arnold, a member of the Hodder Headline Group,
338 Euston Road, London NW1 3BH

http://www.hoddereducation.com

Distributed in the United States of America by
Oxford University Press Inc.,
198 Madison Avenue, New York, NY 10016
Oxford is a registered trademark of Oxford University Press

Whilst the advice and information in this book are believed to be true and
accurate at the date of going to press, neither the authors nor the publisher can
accept any legal responsibility or liability for any errors or omissions that may be
made. In particular (but without limiting the generality of the preceding
disclaimer) every effort has been made to check drug dosages; however, it is still
possible that errors have been missed. Furthermore, dosage schedules are
constantly being revised and new side-effects recognized. For these reasons the
reader is strongly urged to consult the drug companies' printed instructions before
administering any of the drugs recommended in this book.

British Library Cataloguing in Publication Data
A catalogue record for this book is available from the British Library

Library of Congress Cataloging-in-Publication Data
A catalog record for this book is available from the Library of Congress

10-ISBN: 0 340 76319 1
13-ISBN: 978 0 340 76319 3

3 4 5 6 7 8 9 10
Commissioning Editor: Joanna Koster
Project Editor: Wendy Rooke
Production Controller: Deborah Smith
Cover Design: Lee-May Lim

Typeset in 10.5/13 RotisSerif by Charon Tec Pvt. Ltd, Chennai, India
Printed and bound in Italy

What do you think about this book? Or any other Arnold title?
Please visit our website: www.hoddereducation.com

Ο ΜΕΝ ΒΙΟΣ ΒΡΑΧΥΣ, Η ΔΕ ΤΕΧΝΗ ΜΑΚΡΑ, Ο ΔΕ ΚΑΙΡΟΣ
ΟΞΥΣ, Η ΔΕ ΠΕΙΡΑ ΣΦΑΛΕΡΑ, Η ΔΕ ΚΡΙΣΗΣ ΧΑΛΕΠΗ.

ΙΠΠΟΚΡΑΤΗΣ

LIFE IS SHORT, SCIENCE IS LONG; OPPORTUNITY IS ELUSIVE,
EXPERIMENT IS DANGEROUS, JUDGEMENT IS DIFFICULT.

HIPPOCRATES

CONTENTS

PREFACE

Every doctor involved in acute medicine deals with blood
gas or lung function data. Although providing a wealth
of information, much of the content may be lost on the
non-specialist. Frequently the information necessary for
interpretation of basic data is buried deep in heavy specialist
texts. This book sets out to unearth such gems and present
them in a context useful to the frontline doctor. We
accompany the clinical content with underlying physiology,
because we believe that for a little effort it offers worthwhile
enlightenment. As life in clinical medicine is busy, however,
we have placed the physiology in separate sections, so that
those who want the bottom line first can get straight there.

This book is not a technical manual, and details of performing
laboratory tests are not included. Nor is it a reference manual
for the specialist. The aim is to present information that is
accessible to a general medical readership and to bridge the
gap between respiratory physiology and the treatment of
patients.

ACKNOWLEDGEMENTS

We wish to thank Adrian Fineberg and Arlene Jackson for their helpful review of the manuscript from the pulmonary technologist's point of view. A large debt of thanks is owed to Andy Martin who has provided the team with essential IT backup at numerous points along the way.

LIST OF SYMBOLS

Primary symbols (capitals) denoting physical quantities

C   content of a gas in blood
D   diffusing capacity
F   fractional concentration of gas
P   pressure, tension or partial pressure of a gas
Q   volume of blood
R   respiratory exchange ratio
S   saturation of haemoglobin with oxygen
V   volume of a gas
$\cdot$ denotes a time derivative, i.e.
        ventilation $\dot{V}$
        flow $\dot{Q}$
        ventilation–perfusion ratio $\dot{V}/\dot{Q}$
f   denotes respiratory frequency

Secondary symbols denoting location of quantity

In gas phase (small capitals)

A   aveolar gas
D   dead space gas
E   expired gas
I   inspired gas
T   tidal

In blood (lower case)

a   arterial blood
c   capillary blood
v   venous blood
s   shunt
t   total

Adding $^-$ denotes mean or mixed, i.e. mixed venous blood $\bar{v}$
Adding $'$ denotes end, i.e. capillary blood c'

LIST OF ABBREVIATIONS

ABG	arterial blood gases
ALI	acute lung injury
ARDS	acute respiratory distress syndrome
CC	closing capacity
CFA	cryptogenic fibrosing alveolitis
C_L	compliance of the lung
CO	carbon monoxide
COPD	chronic obstructive pulmonary disease
CPAP	continuous positive airway pressure
C_{RS}	compliance of the combined respiratory system
CT	computed tomography
CV	closing volume
C_W	compliance of the chest wall
EAA	extrinsic allergic alveolitis
FET	forced expiratory time
FEV_1	forced expiratory volume in 1 second
F_IO_2	fractional concentration of oxygen inspired
FRC	functional residual capacity
FVC	forced vital capacity
Hb	haemoglobin concentration
K_{CO}	transfer coefficient
MEF_{50}	maximum expiratory flow at 50% of forced vital capacity
MEFV	maximum expiratory flow volume
MIF_{50}	maximum inspiratory flow at 50% of forced vital capacity

MIFV	maximum inspiratory flow volume
P_aCO_2	partial pressure of carbon dioxide in arterial blood
P_ACO_2	partial pressure of carbon dioxide in alveolar gas
P_aO_2	partial pressure of oxygen in arterial blood
P_AO_2	partial pressure of oxygen in alveolar gas
PCO_2	partial pressure of carbon dioxide
$P\bar{E}CO_2$	partial pressure of carbon dioxide in mixed expiratory gas
PEEP	positive end-expiratory pressure
PEF	peak expiratory flow
P_IO_2	partial pressure of inspired oxygen
PO_2	partial pressure of oxygen
$\dot{Q}$	perfusion
RV	residual volume
SLE	systemic lupus erythematosus
TLC	total lung capacity
TL_{CO}	transfer capacity of the lung for carbon monoxide
$\dot{V}$	ventilation
V_A	alveolar volume
VC	vital capacity
$\dot{V}_E$	minute volume
V_r	relaxation volume
V_T	tidal volume

TESTS OF MECHANICAL PROPERTIES

PEAK EXPIRATORY FLOW

Key definition

● PEF Peak expiratory flow. Maximum flow achieved during an expiration delivered with maximal force from total lung capacity.

Physiology: peak expiratory flow

The peak expiratory flow is the highest airflow velocity transiently achieved during a forced expiration. It is a contrived test, as at no time, even in extreme breathlessness does anyone take such a breath. But, because flow is a function of airway resistance, and the majority of resistance is encountered in the upper airway, PEF is an excellent indicator of large airway patency.

As well as airway resistance, peak flow is a function of lung recoil, which increases as the lung is inflated. Measurements should, therefore, always be made after a full inspiration.

WHY MEASURE PEAK FLOW?

The peak flow is a good indicator of asthmatic control. No asthmatic should be without a mini peak flow meter, and familiarity of their own normal range of values.

Many asthmatic patients have little sensation of increased airways resistance. So-called 'poor perceivers' may have no awareness of a falling PEF until the drop is catastrophic. The peak flow meter gives an objective and early indication of the need to increase therapy or seek help.

PITFALL

An isolated peak flow reading has no value in diagnosing the cause of respiratory insufficiency.

VARIABILITY

Diurnal variation in PEF is a cardinal feature of asthma. Greater than 20% difference between the highest and lowest daily readings in the appropriate clinical setting is diagnostic of asthma. The dip in PEF is usually in the early morning or late at night (Fig. 1.1).

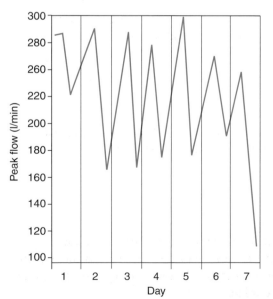

Fig. 1.1

Diurnal peak flow variability

Peak flow only has a slight diurnal variation in normal subjects, with the lowest values usually seen in the early hours of the morning. The wide variation in this asthmatic is seen when under very poor control, ending with a final plummet.

- Peak flow should be measured at home by asthmatics morning and night, and may be charted in a PEF diary.
- Lack of variability of PEF in a smoker with an obstructive defect supports a diagnosis of chronic obstructive pulmonary disease (COPD).

CLINICAL ASPECTS OF PEF: ASSESSMENT OF ASTHMA SEVERITY

- In a patient with asthma, a PEF of less than 50% predicted (or the patient's normal best, whichever is less) is a feature of acute severe asthma. A patient with a PEF of this order, particularly when this persists after bronchodilator therapy, will need hospital admission.
- A peak flow of 33% predicted (or patient's best) is a feature of life-threatening asthma.
- Wide diurnal swings PEF are a feature of asthma under poor control (Fig. 1.1). Large variation in PEF is also found in the recovery phase of acute severe asthma and indicates ongoing lability. A patient who has been admitted to hospital with acute asthma should not be discharged until the diurnal variation of PEF is less than 25%.

PITFALL

Diurnal variability may be missed if PEF is not measured first thing in the morning, prior to bronchodilator treatment.

TECHNIQUE

The subject is to take a hard short puff after a maximal inspiration, as though blowing candles out. It is not necessary to continue blowing until empty. Three readings are taken and the highest value recorded.

TYPICAL VALUES

These are read off standard charts.

See Fig. 1.2.

Typical predicted values of PEF:

- Male Caucasian, aged 30, height 6ft (184 cm): 650 l/min
- Female Caucasian, aged 60, height 5ft 4in (163 cm): 440 l/min.

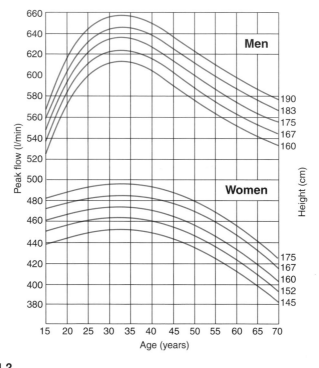

Fig. 1.2

Peak expiratory flow in normal subjects

During childhood, peak flows are the same for boys as girls of the same height. During adolescence the two groups diverge, so that the predicted PEF for a short man is greater than that of a tall woman. Hence the two sets of curves have no overlap. (Reproduced from Gregg, I. and Nunn, A. J. 1973: Peak expiratory flow in normal subjects. *Br Med J* 3(5874):282–4, with permission from the BMJ Publishing Group.)

KEYPOINTS

- Diurnal variability in PEF is the hallmark of asthma.
- Peak flow measurements are essential in managing asthma to predict exacerbation, assess severity and chart recovery.
- There are many causes of low PEF other than asthma. Peak flow is not a diagnostic test, and a low reading should prompt further investigation.

2

SPIROMETRY

Spirometry is one of the most widely used lung function tests. The spirogram is a plot of the volume/time curve (Fig. 2.1) and the basic values used to interpret spirometry are the FVC, FEV_1, FEV_1/FVC ratio.

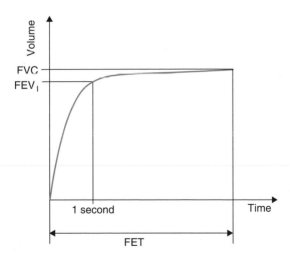

Fig. 2.1

Normal spirogram

Anatomy of the spirogram. The maximum value obtained is the forced vital capacity. A normal subject should be able to expel this volume in 3–4 sec (forced expiratory time, FET). There should be a fairly sharp bend or 'elbow' in the curve around 1 sec before it flattens out as flow reduces and the lung empties. The ratio of FEV_1 to FVC should be >0.7.

Key definitions

- FVC Forced vital capacity
  Total volume expelled by a forced exhalation from a maximal inspiration.
- VC Vital capacity
  Total volume expelled by a slow exhalation from a maximal inspiration.
- FEV_1 Forced expiratory volume in 1 second
  Volume exhaled in the first second of an FVC manoeuvre.
- FET Forced expiratory time
  Time taken for a subject to exhale their vital capacity in a forced expiration.

Physiology: spirometry in restrictive and obstructive defects

VC and FEV_1 are both volumetric measurements, but as a volume expired within a set time, FEV_1 is a reflection of the *speed of emptying* of the lung and, therefore, indirectly *airflow*. The FEV_1/FVC ratio can be considered as a ratio of flow/volume.

The lung is a spring that recoils to cause expiration. Forced expiratory flows are a function of the lung's recoil and the total lung capacity, as well as airway patency and to a lesser extent muscle strength. (See 'Forced expiratory flows' in Chapter 9 'Airway Resistance' to understand why recoil is more important than muscle strength in determining maximum expiratory airflow.)

Restrictive disorders are those in which expansion of the lung is restricted, either due to loss of alveolar volume, or diseases of the chest wall, pleura or neuromuscular apparatus. Maximal flow depends on the volume of lung generating it, and so reduction in total lung capacity reduces the peak expiratory flow and FEV_1 that can be attained. In *restrictive* disorders, FEV_1 is reduced in proportion to the loss of lung volume, so that the FEV_1/FVC ratio is maintained (Fig. 2.2).

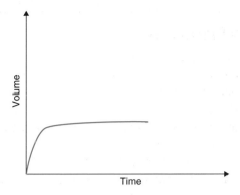

Fig. 2.2

Spirogram in restrictive lung disease

The curve is of normal shape and proportions, but reduced in size.

Airway disease affects flow *more* than volume; i.e. the lung empties more slowly. These disorders are described as *obstructive*. Accordingly, FEV_1 is reduced to a greater extent than the FVC, and the FEV_1/FVC ratio is reduced (Fig. 2.3).

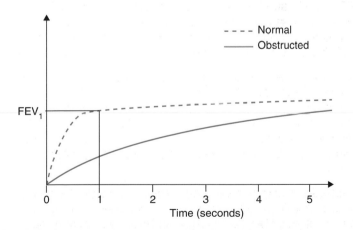

Fig. 2.3

Spirogram in obstructive lung disease

The vital capacity in this subject is only slightly reduced. The FEV_1, however, is greatly diminished, giving a much-reduced FEV_1/FVC ratio.

> **KEYPOINTS**
>
> ● Increasing expiratory effort increases airflow up to a point, but a plateau is reached above which further effort brings no increase in flow. Beyond this point, flow is dependent on the lung's mechanical properties, making the FEV_1 highly reproducible.
> ● Spirometry is the most important estimate of lung function and should be measured at presentation and followed in all respiratory patients.

What extra information does spirometry give in comparison to peak flow?

● The FEV_1/FVC ratio is central in the initial assessment, as it categorizes the respiratory disorders into obstructive or restrictive.
● PEF is not affected in the early stages of a restrictive disorder.
● Reproducibility of spirometry is better than peak flow, as peak flow is more effort dependent.

SPIROMETRY IN OBSTRUCTIVE DISORDERS

See Figs 2.3–2.5.

● $FEV_1/FVC < 0.7$ is diagnostic of obstruction. This is caused by airways disease, the usual causes being chronic bronchitis, emphysema and asthma. Less common causes of an obstructive defect include bronchiectasis, obliterative bronchiolitis and cryptogenic organizing pneumonia (COP)/bronchiolitis obliterans and organizing pneumonitis (BOOP).
● The severity of an obstructive disorder is measured by the reduction of FEV_1 in comparison to predicted.

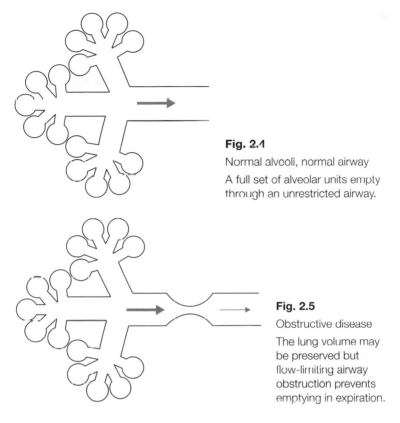

Fig. 2.4

Normal alveoli, normal airway

A full set of alveolar units empty through an unrestricted airway.

Fig. 2.5

Obstructive disease

The lung volume may be preserved but flow-limiting airway obstruction prevents emptying in expiration.

- The absolute value of FEV_1 is the best predictor of survival in COPD and probably the most important single variable in respiratory medicine.
- PEF is relatively preserved in comparison to FEV_1 in severe COPD, and so tends to underestimate disease progression. FEV_1 is a better measurement to assess severity in airways disease.

PITFALL

If FEV_1/FVC is greater than 0.7, the diagnosis is unlikely to be COPD.

Spirometry in emphysema

In pure emphysema (without bronchitis), there is no physical intraluminal obstruction. Tissue destruction causes loss of lung parenchyma distal to the terminal bronchiole. The loss of tissue in which the airways are embedded results in their collapse during expiration, causing a functional obstruction (see Chapter 9 'Airway resistance').

Is there any relationship between PEF and FEV_1?

FEV_1 and peak flow both reflect flow, and so, not surprisingly, a linear relationship has been found in both normal subjects and subjects with obstructive disease.

● In chronic airflow limitation, PEF is approximately proportional to FEV_1, with the PEF (in l/min) being approximately equal to $150 \times FEV_1$ (in l).

Straight line spirogram

See Fig. 2.6. In large airway obstruction, PEF is affected more than FEV_1. A reduction of the PEF/FEV_1 ratio to less than 100 is suggestive of a large airway lesion. The ascent of the spirogram is dampened, causing a *straight line spirogram*. The flow-volume loop, however, is a better means of demonstrating a large airway obstruction.

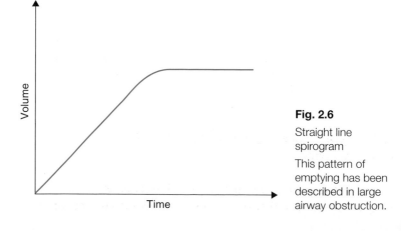

Fig. 2.6

Straight line spirogram

This pattern of emptying has been described in large airway obstruction.

Forced expiratory time (FET)

Forced expiratory time is the time taken for a subject to exhale their vital capacity in a forced expiration. A subject with normal airways can exhale the vital capacity in 3 sec. Where severe airflow limitation exists 15 sec or longer may be needed.

Some older mechanical spirometers record a spirogram for only the first 6 sec of expiration (Fig. 2.7). If measurement is stopped at this stage, a falsely low FVC and, therefore, falsely high FEV_1/FVC will be recorded. This problem is avoided by instructing the subject to keep blowing until empty, *even after the pen has reached the edge of the recording paper,* so it continues to register volume.

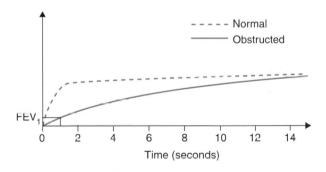

Fig. 2.7

Spirogram in severe obstructive airways disease

In this severely obstructed spirogram, the vital capacity measured at 14 sec is still relatively well preserved. Had it been measured at 6 sec, a falsely low reading would have been made, giving a misleading FEV_1/FVC ratio. The forced expiratory time here is around 14 sec.

SPIROMETRY IN RESTRICTIVE DISORDERS

Restrictive disorders are those in which expansion of the lung is restricted, either due to loss of alveolar volume, or diseases of the chest wall, pleura or neuromuscular apparatus. A space-occupying lesion elsewhere in the thorax that impinges on the lung expansion also causes a restrictive problem.

A restrictive defect is characterized physiologically by a reduction in total lung capacity, but may be inferred by a reduction in vital capacity in the presence of a proportionate reduction of FEV_1. The resulting spirogram is of normal shape but reduced amplitude.

Lung diseases causing a restrictive defect

See Fig. 2.2. A restrictive defect is seen in the diffuse lung diseases, where obliteration of alveolar units causes a reduction of total lung capacity (TLC; Table 2.1).

Table 2.1 Diffuse lung diseases associated with restrictive disorders

Condition	Examples
Extrinsic allergic alveolitis	Farmer's lung, bird fancier's lung
Pneumoconioses	Coal worker's pneumoconiosis, asbestosis
Collagen vascular diseases	Scleroderma, rheumatoid, polymyositis, Sjorgren's syndrome
Sarcoid	
Cryptogenic fibrosing alveolitis	
Toxins	Paraquat ingestion
Drug damage	Amiodarone, methotrexate, bleomycin
Radiotherapy	

- Loss of lung volume defines the restrictive state and TLC directly measures this. FVC, however, reflects the TLC, and is a convenient and useful means of monitoring response/progression in diffuse lung disease, along with TLC and TL_{CO}.
- If the lung is small and stiff, as in interstitial lung disease, the lung may have greater recoil than would be expected for its volume. Here the FEV_1/FVC ratio may be high.

Other intrathoracic causes of a restrictive defect

Because FEV_1 and FVC depend on lung volume, a restrictive picture is seen in any cause of a reduced TLC (Table 2.2).

Table 2.2 Other intrathoracic causes of a restrictive defect

Condition	Examples
Post-surgical	Pneumonectomy, lobectomy
Space-occupying lesion	Hiatus hernia, gross cardiomegaly, pleural effusion

Disorders of the thoracic wall

See also Chapter 8 'Respiratory Muscle Power'. Diseases of the chest wall also reduce the maximum available lung capacity causing a restrictive defect (extrapulmonary restriction). For causes, see Table 2.3.

Table 2.3 Thoracic wall problems causing a restrictive disorder

Condition	Examples
Pleural disease	Pleural encasement (e.g. post-empyema)
Skeletal	Ankylosing spondylitis, thoracoplasty
Obesity	
Neuromuscular disorder	Motor neurone disease, Guillain–Barré, bilateral diaphragmatic paralysis, muscular dystrophy, myopathy See Chapter 8 'Respiratory Muscle Power'
Severe dermatological disease	Scleroderma, circumferential burns

● Obesity is a common cause of a mild restrictive defect.

TECHNIQUE

Vital capacity (VC) is measured by asking the patient to exhale after a full deep inspiration (total lung capacity, TLC) until there is no breath left in their lungs (residual volume, RV).

An FVC measurement is performed by repeating the above, but exhaling as hard and as quickly as possible. Three attempts should be made at this manoeuvre, during which two FEV_1 values within 5% or 100 ml of the best should be obtained. Widely varying readings taken on the same occasion suggest either bad technique or that the subject is not fully cooperative.

The shape of the graph is easier to interpret instantly than paired numerical values, and the smoothness of the curve confirms that it is free from artefact. It should be possible to superimpose the plots from successive attempts to check consistency. There are digital meters available that produce the numerical values only, but these are unsuitable for making a diagnosis. Hand-held digital meters are useful for assessing recovery from acute exacerbations on the ward or monitoring progression in the clinic.

Measurement should be compared to normal values, standardized for gender, height and age, and expressed as a percentage predicted. Computerized systems automatically perform this calculation. Non-Caucasians have lower predicted values than Caucasians. The normal range quoted encompasses 95% of the healthy, normal population.

TYPICAL VALUES

Male, aged 20, height 6 ft (184 cm): $FEV_1/FVC = 5.0/6.0$ l.
Female, aged 60, height 5 ft 6 in (169 cm):
$FEV_1/FVC = 2.7/3.5$ l.

- An FEV_1 of less than a litre is a major impairment.
- An FEV_1 of 0.4 l is about as low as it tends to get and indicates end-stage lung disease.
- FEV_1/FVC is normally greater than 0.75; it may be up to 0.9 in teenagers, and may drop to 0.7 in the fit elderly.

PITFALL

Be wary of attributing respiratory failure to COPD if the FEV_1 is greater that 1 l. An alternative cause should be sought.

Summary

FEV$_1$ reflects airflow. Used for monitoring airway disease, i.e. COPD and asthma.
FVC and VC Used for monitoring restrictive disease and neuromuscular weakness.

Obstructive disorder: FEV$_1$/FVC < 0.7.
Pathophysiology: airway disease causing airflow limitation that slows lung emptying.

Restrictive disorder: FEV$_1$/FVC normal or high.
Pathophysiology: reduced lung filling causing proportionate reduction in airflow.

3

AIRWAY RESPONSIVENESS TESTING

There are two types of test: bronchodilator and bronchial hyper-responsiveness testing.

BRONCHODILATOR TESTING

Spirometry is performed before and after administration of bronchodilator. FEV_1 is the preferred measurement because of its reproducibility. An increase of 12% *and* 200 ml in either FEV_1 or FVC provides evidence of reversibility[1].

Should reversibility testing be performed if initial spirometry is normal?

The range of normality is quite wide; therefore, a patient may have an FEV_1 of 10% above predicted before losing 20% of their FEV_1 to bronchospasm, leaving a value of 90% predicted. This would still lie within the normal range however. A bronchodilator test under these circumstances may restore 90% to 110% and thereby unmask significant bronchoconstriction.

---

[1] American Thoracic Society. Lung function testing: selection of normal values and interpretive strategies. *American Review of Respiratory Disease* 1991; 144: 1202–1218. Available at http://www.thoracic.org/adobe/statements/lftvalue1-17.pdf.

● Reversibility should be assessed in all cases of presumed COPD and asthma. COPD frequently has a component of reversibility, which should be sought and treated.

PITFALL

Reversibility leading to restoration of normal values does not occur in COPD but confirms a diagnosis of asthma. COPD should not be diagnosed if normal spirometry is attainable.

Why perform bronchodilator tests if the diagnosis of COPD is already established?

Failure to measure lung function after bronchodilatation in COPD or asthma may lead to a large underestimation of best respiratory function. This is likely to result in undertreatment.

A positive response to a trial justifies the long-term prescription of inhaled steroid. Presence of significant reversibility on steroid treatment implies that there is scope for a higher dose. *Significant reversibility may occur even in severe COPD.*

A negative bronchodilator reversibility test at any severity of disease does not preclude a subjective improvement in breathlessness or exercise tolerance with therapy.

TECHNIQUE: BRONCHODILATOR TESTING

Patients should not have taken short-acting β agonist for the preceding 4–8 hours, long-acting agonist or slow-release aminophylline for 24 hours. Testing should be performed when the subject is well.

FEV_1 should be measured before and 20 minutes after inhaled or nebulized β agonist; or before and 45 minutes after nebulized ipratroprium (or both in combination).

BRONCHIAL HYPER-RESPONSIVENESS TESTING

Key definitions

FEV_1 PD_{20} Provocation dose of bronchoconstrictor required to provoke a reduction in FEV_1 of 20%

FEV_1 PC_{20} Provocation concentration of bronchoconstrictor required to provoke a reduction in FEV_1 of 20%

These tests measure the response of the airways to agents known to cause bronchoconstriction, such as histamine or methacholine.

A limited bronchoconstrictor response is seen in normal subjects, but this is greatly exaggerated in asthmatics. A positive response is indicative of airway *hyper-responsiveness*, rather than asthma *per se*. This may also occur in chronic bronchitis, recovery from respiratory tract infection, left ventricular failure, asymptomatic smokers and 5% of otherwise normal subjects.

Bronchial responsiveness testing may be useful in making a positive diagnosis of asthma in subjects with infrequent attacks, who present to the clinic when normal. Home peak-flow monitoring is generally preferred because it gives the patient greater insight into their own PEF variability.

Applications include the following:

Excluding asthma
A normal bronchial provocation test to histamine virtually excludes asthma.

Chronic non-productive cough
Bronchial provocation may be useful in patients with chronic non-productive cough, which may be due to asthma even if

the patient does not complain of wheeze. A positive histamine challenge test would support a diagnosis of asthma.

Technique

This is performed with increasing doses of inhaled histamine or methacholine. The dose required to provoke a fall in FEV_1 of 20% is found by interpolation. Bronchodilators should be withheld for 6 hours previously, cromoglycate for 12 hours and antihistamines and leukotriene antagonists for 48 hours.

Airways resistance or conductance may be used as a more sensitive measure of response than FEV_1.

● Severe reactions are rare, but facilities to resuscitate should be available. Absolute contraindications include recent severe asthma, FEV_1 <1.2 l, recent myocardial infarction or stroke.

Typical values

PD_{20} is normally greater than 4 μmol histamine.
PC_{20} is normally greater than 8 mg/ml histamine.

4

THE FLOW VOLUME LOOP

The subject performs an FVC manoeuvre, but when residual volume is reached (at the end of expiration) a sharp full inspiratory breath is taken, back up to total lung capacity. The resultant graph has a positive and negative phase of flow: the maximum expiratory flow volume (MEFV) and maximum inspiratory flow volume (MIFV) curves. The two form a continuous loop (Fig. 4.1; see p. 26).

The graph is a plot of maximal flow (in differential terms rate of change of volume) against volume. Each point on the graph is the maximal flow for that lung volume. There is no indication of time on the record.

MEASURABLE PARAMETERS

Maximum expiratory flows (MEFs)

See Fig. 4.2, p. 27. The following parameters are derived from the maximum expiratory flow curve, along with PEF. Only PEF is widely quoted as a stand-alone test, however.

- MEF_{75} Maximal flow at 75% of VC
- MEF_{50} Maximal flow at 50% of VC
- MEF_{25} Maximal flow at 25% of VC

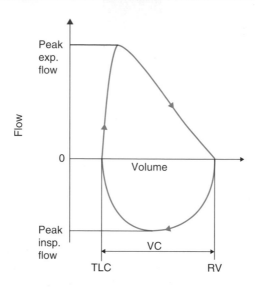

Fig. 4.1

Normal flow volume loop

Anatomy of the flow volume loop. The essential form of the flow volume loop is a skewed triangle on top of a semicircle. Above the *x* axis is the maximum expiratory flow volume curve; below is the maximum inspiratory flow volume curve. The subject takes a full breath to TLC before starting. On commencement of expiration (at the origin), flow should rise steeply to the peak flow and then fall along a linear path until no more air can be expelled. At residual volume, a sharp inspiration is taken back to TLC. The loop is conventionally pictured this way, with the *x* axis decreasing in value from left to right. The peak inspiratory flow is usually about three-quarters of the value of the peak expiratory flow. The normal loop, therefore, rises further up above the *x* axis than it dips below.

Maximum inspiratory flow (MIF)

See Fig. 4.3, p. 27.

- MIF_{50} Maximum inspiratory flow during the inspiratory phase. This is normally equal to or slightly greater than MEF_{50}.

What advantage does the flow volume loop have over spirometry?

The flow volume loop generally supplements spirometry but provides additional information

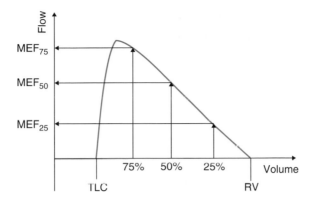

Fig. 4.2

Maximum expiratory flows

The flow rates at 75%, 50% and 25% of vital capacity may be quoted. The MEF_{25} is on the point of the curve that is most affected by airway obstruction and is, therefore, a sensitive indicator of an asthmatic tendency or early emphysema. The normal range is wide, however, and it is always better to look at the curve, and see whether the descending section of the expiratory curve is straight as it should be or tending to concavity, indicative of airflow obstruction.

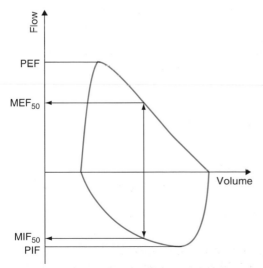

Fig. 4.3

Maximal inspiratory flows

The peak inspiratory flow is generally about 75% of the peak expiratory flow. However, the expiratory flow rate at half vital capacity is approximately equal to the inspiratory flow rate at the same point, i.e. $MIF_{50} = MEF_{50}$. Alteration of this ratio is suggestive of airway obstruction. The asymmetry seen in the inspiratory curve is a normal variant.

in certain circumstances:

- The shape of the normal curve is sensitive to airway obstruction, showing early changes in COPD. FEV_1 is relatively insensitive in detection of early disease, as FEV_1/FVC varies with age.
- The flow volume loop has characteristic patterns in large airway obstruction and respiratory muscle weakness.

NB: No measurement of vital capacity is made during a flow volume loop manoeuvre. This should be separately recorded.

PATTERNS OF ABNORMALITY

Reduced pattern

See Fig. 4.4. This is seen if the lungs and respiratory muscles are normal, but the total lung capacity reduced for some other reason. The flow volume loop is of normal shape but reduced amplitude. Such a pattern is seen post pneumonectomy or lobectomy, or in the presence of pleural effusions large enough to reduce TLC significantly.

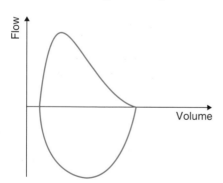

Fig. 4.4

Reduced flow volume curve

This curve was taken from a 45-year-old with normal lungs but large bilateral pleural effusions. The form of the curve is normal but the size is reduced proportionately throughout, owing to the reduction in TLC (and vital capacity).

Airflow limitation

See Figs 4.5–4.7; pp. 29–30. The terminal portion of the expiratory loop, i.e. beyond the MEF_{25}, is relatively independent of effort (see 'Forced expiratory flows' in Chapter 9 'Airway resistance'). The characteristic abnormality

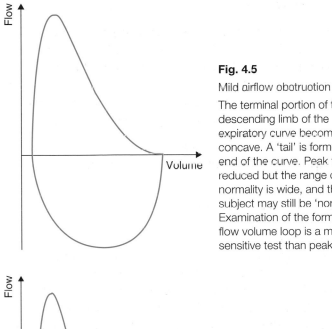

Fig. 4.5

Mild airflow obstruction

The terminal portion of the descending limb of the expiratory curve becomes concave. A 'tail' is formed on the end of the curve. Peak flow is reduced but the range of normality is wide, and this subject may still be 'normal'. Examination of the form of the flow volume loop is a more sensitive test than peak flow.

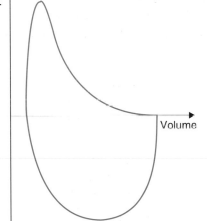

Fig. 4.6

Moderate airflow obstruction

As airflow obstruction progresses, the expiratory curve becomes concave throughout and the peak expiratory flow falls. Consequently, the height of the expiratory curve falls in relation to that of the inspiratory curve.

in airways disease is concavity of this normally linear region, corresponding to airway closure (Fig. 4.5).

This may be the most sensitive indicator of asthma or early airway disease, especially in the young fit patient whose spirometric values remain comfortably within the normal

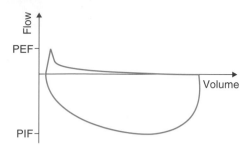

Fig. 4.7

Severe airflow obstruction

In severe airflow limitation, the flow rate collapses soon after peak flow due to airway closure. The peak expiratory flow itself is greatly reduced and small in comparison to PIF.

range. It may be useful for detecting exercise-induced asthma, if a recording is performed before and after exertion, so a subject acts as their own normal reference.

Large airway obstruction

This may be considered as:

Extrathoracic airway obstruction (see Fig. 4.8; p. 31)

The *extra*thoracic airway tends to collapse in *in*spiration, when the luminal pressure is less than atmospheric. An obstructing lesion sited here would cause greater limitation of the MIFV curve.

This may be caused by vocal cord paralysis (post thyroidectomy, motor neurone disease), extrinsic compression from a cervical lesion (tumour, goitre),or a tracheal lesion above the sternal notch, e.g. a tumour or stricture.

Intrathoracic airway obstruction (see Fig. 4.9; p. 32)

A forced expiration reduces the calibre of intrathoracic airways as the positive pleural pressure is transmitted to the airways (Fig. 4.10; see p. 32). An *intra*thoracic obstructing lesion would further reduce airway patency during expiration, with a characteristic effect on the MEFV curve. The greatest attenuation is seen during early expiration around peak flow.

This may be caused by extrinsic compression from a mediastinal mass, e.g. retrosternal goitre or a tracheal lesion below the sternal notch.

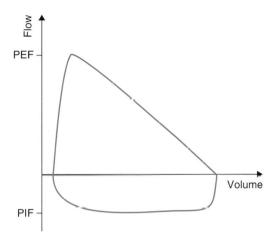

Fig. 4.8

Extrathoracic obstruction

The inspiratory curve is flattened with substantial reduction of the PIF.
The pressure within the airways is always negative during inspiration, so the airways have a continuous tendency to collapse. Within the thorax the airways are held open by the expanding force generated by the inspiratory muscles.

In the extrathoracic trachea, only the cartilaginous rings maintain patency and there is normally a reduction of the diameter of the trachea on inspiration.

If there is extrathoracic large-airway obstruction, when the lumen narrows in inspiration the walls of the airway approximate around the site of the narrowing, with resultant airflow limitation around it. Inspiratory flow is reduced in comparison to expiratory flow.

Fixed airway obstruction (see Fig. 4.11; p. 33)

It is possible that an obstruction may rigidly narrow the airway. Wherever it is sited, this will provide a fixed limitation to flow in both phases of respiration.

Restrictive pulmonary disorders

The first change seen is a reduction in vital capacity (Fig. 4.12; see p. 33). In interstitial lung disease, there is an increase in the stiffness of the lung, which provides greater recoil in expiration. Consequently, peak flow rate is maintained at first, despite loss of volume.

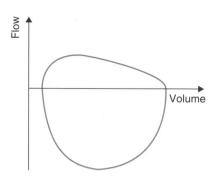

Fig. 4.9

Intrathoracic obstruction

There is flattening of the expiratory curve and reduction in the peak expiratory flow. Peak flow occurs late in the course of expiration. During expiration, the compressive effect of positive pleural pressure narrows intrathoracic airways. Any luminal lesion within the large airway severely compromises the expiratory flow. During inspiration, the diameter of intrathoracic airways is increased and the reduction of flow during this phase less noticeable.

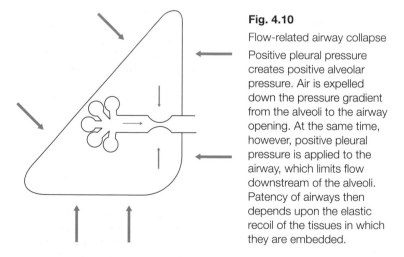

Fig. 4.10

Flow-related airway collapse

Positive pleural pressure creates positive alveolar pressure. Air is expelled down the pressure gradient from the alveoli to the airway opening. At the same time, however, positive pleural pressure is applied to the airway, which limits flow downstream of the alveoli. Patency of airways then depends upon the elastic recoil of the tissues in which they are embedded.

The effect of increased recoil on the expiratory flow curve is a steepening of the slope of the descending limb, from the same peak flow, to residual volume. The steepening of descent may even progress to convexity of the descending segment (Fig. 4.13; see p. 33).

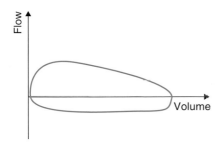

Fig. 4.11

Fixed large airway obstruction

A large airway obstruction may rigidly narrow the wall, so that no variation in diameter occurs with respiration. This causes significant reduction in flow throughout inspiration and expiration.

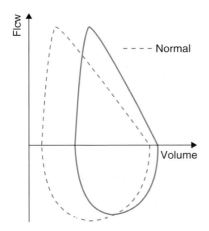

- - - - Normal

Fig. 4.12

Early pulmonary restrictive defect

There is loss of vital capacity and steepening of the descending limb of the expiratory curve. The increased lung recoil maintains peak expiratory flow in mild disease, despite the loss of vital capacity on which it depends.

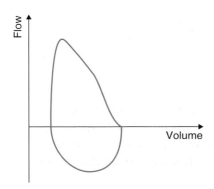

Fig. 4.13

Moderate restriction

There is loss of vital capacity and peak flow. Convexity of the descending limb of the expiratory curve may be seen. This is in contrast to chronic airflow obstruction, and indicates better lung emptying and flow than would be predicted for the corresponding volume, owing to the increased lung recoil.

With disease progression, peak flow and the amplitude of the whole loop are reduced (Fig. 4.14).

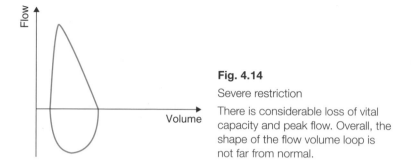

Fig. 4.14

Severe restriction

There is considerable loss of vital capacity and peak flow. Overall, the shape of the flow volume loop is not far from normal.

The TLC and RV are both also reduced, so that the whole loop is theoretically shifted to the right (Fig. 4.12). However, as these parameters are not measurable by this means, they are not displayed.

Neuromuscular disease

When there is weakness of the chest wall musculature (extrapulmonary restriction), the flow volume loop produces a pattern which is distinct from that of restrictive pulmonary disease.

Generalized muscle weakness (see Fig. 4.15; p. 35)

The peak flow occurs later in expiration, with a gentler rise of the expiratory curve. Because inspiratory flow is more effort dependent, muscular weakness causes relatively greater reduction in the amplitude of the MIF curve, with corresponding decrease in MIF_{50}.

Saw-tooth curve (see Fig. 4.16; p. 35)

Reproducible spikes may occur in all individuals, probably corresponding to subsegmental opening and closure. A more pronounced and non-reproducible pattern may be seen in a variety of neurological conditions, particularly those associated with dystonia, including bulbar muscle weakness and

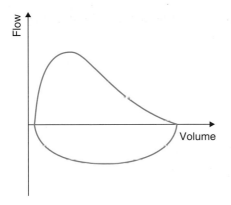

Fig. 4.15

Respiratory muscle weakness

The ascent of the curve to peak expiratory flow is gentle instead of the usual steep climb. The peak flow itself is reduced and delayed. The most effort-dependent part of the respiratory cycle is inspiration, and there is a proportionately greater reduction in inspiratory flow rates. MEF_{50} is greater than the MIF_{50}.

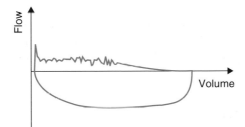

Fig. 4.16

'Saw-tooth curve'

This flow volume loop was taken from a 30-year-old with polychondritis. There is instability in the expiratory curve. This is due to closure of intrathoracic airways because the cartilage is unable to maintain airway patency under the positive pressure of a forced expiration. There may be similar oscillations elsewhere on the curve.

extrapyramidal disorder. It may also be seen in subjects with obstructive sleep apnoea, upper airway stenosis and after thermal injury to the airway.

Pharyngeal notch (see Fig. 4.17; p. 36)

There may be complete collapse of the pharynx in inspiration. This causes notching of the inspiratory segment. The same pattern may occur in subjects with vocal cord dysfunction. It may be seen in anyone with poor coordination of the upper

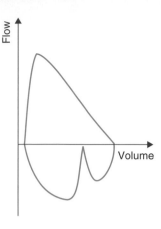

Fig. 4.17

Pharyngeal notch

Control of the pharyngeal musculature is necessary during the forced inspiratory manoeuvre to prevent collapse under the negative pressure. If there is weakness here as in bulbar palsy, a characteristic notch may be seen. This may also occur with vocal cord dysfunction. A similar pattern may be seen on a subject's first attempt before they are practised in maintaining upper airway patency during this unnatural manoeuvre.

airway muscles, including normal subjects with poor technique. This may occur repeatedly as an oscillation, causing the pattern of pharyngeal flutter, associated with a narrow pharynx.

Summary

- Obstructive disorder: concavity of descending limb of expiratory curve.
- Restrictive disorder: steepening of descent of expiratory curve, followed by reduction in amplitude of loop, but preservation of shape.
- Extrathoracic airway obstruction: flattening of inspiratory curve.
- Intrathoracic large airway obstruction: flattening of expiratory curve.

5

STATIC COMPLIANCE

Key definitions
- C_L Static compliance of the lung
- C_W Static compliance of the chest wall
- C_{RS} Combined static compliance of the lung and chest wall (respiratory system)

Compliance is the change in volume per change in inflation pressure. It is a measure of the distensibility of the lung and chest wall, which is inversely related to elastic recoil.

The force exerted by the inspiratory muscles in inflating the lungs is greater than the recoil alone. This additional impedance is airway resistance, which originates from friction between air and mucosa. Compliance studies are, therefore, conducted under static conditions, i.e. during breath-holding.

Approximately half of the work of breathing is expended against the elastic recoil of the lungs and chest wall, and remains in the system as potential energy, to be released in the next expiration. Half the work done is against resistive airway forces and is lost by dissipation as heat.

Physiology: compliance
The volume of air held in the lung at TLC, FRC and RV is governed by the elastic properties of the lung and chest wall. Studies of these properties have been conducted using an isolated

cadaveric preparations, so that the lung and chest wall could be separated from each other. The isolated lung is inflated to capacity and progressively deflated through a range of volumes, at which airway pressure is measured under static conditions.

In this way, a pressure/volume curve may be plotted for the lung (Fig. 5.1). Compliance is the slope of the curve.

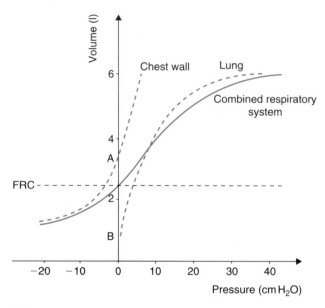

Fig. 5.1

Deflation pressure volume curve for the components of compliance of the respiratory system

The graph indicates the volume occupied by the thoracic cavity and lungs at a range of airway pressures during deflation. Negative pressures (suction) are needed to reduce volume further than the relaxation volume.

At zero pressure, the chest wall assumes a volume (A) greater than does the isolated lung (B). The relaxation volume of the combined intact system is between the two. This volume is FRC. At this point the lungs tend to contract and the chest wall to expand, with a resultant negative pleural pressure. Compliance at a particular volume is given by the gradient of the curve at that volume. Compliance (the gradient of) the combined curve is seen to be less than either of the components.

The compliance is seen to decrease as the lung expands, i.e. it gets stiffer as it gets fuller.

By inflating the empty thorax a similar graph can be constructed for the chest wall in isolation. The curve for the combined respiratory system is the sum of component pressures at each volume.

The two curves represent the compliance of the chest wall (C_W) and lung (C_L), respectively. The intercept of each with the y axis corresponds to the volume taken up when no inflation pressure is applied, i.e. the relaxation volume. For the chest wall, this is greater than the lung. Therefore, when the two are separated, they tend to spring apart, to their own neutral states. When coupled together *in situ*, an in-between volume is assumed, which is then the relaxation volume of the combined respiratory system (V_r). The compliance curve for the combined system (C_{RS}) is indicated by the solid line.

Because the slope of the curve varies along its course, compliance is usually quoted at functional residual capacity (FRC). The recoil pressure of the lung originates from the elasticity of the parenchyma and the surface tension of tissue fluid. The latter is much-reduced by surfactant.

CONTRIBUTORS TO COMBINED COMPLIANCE

Chest wall compliance and lung compliance normally each make an equal contribution to the total. In children, the chest wall is far more compliant, so most of the total stiffness of the respiratory system is due to the lung itself.

Lung compliance

- Increased lung compliance (reduced recoil) is found in emphysema.
- Reduced compliance (increased recoil) is seen in interstitial lung disease, any cause of pulmonary venous congestion or

pulmonary oedema, and most dramatically in the acute respiratory distress syndrome (ARDS).

Chest wall compliance

A reduction in chest wall compliance may be caused by pleural thickening and skeletal disorders, such as kyphoscoliosis and ankylosing spondylitis. Dermatological conditions may have the same effect, as in the 'hide-bound chest' of scleroderma. Rarely, circumferential chest wall burns with eschar formation may reduce compliance enough to necessitate urgent surgical release (escharotomy).

The diaphragm is splinted if abdominal pressure is raised, so that compliance is reduced in obesity, pregnancy, ascites and massive intra-abdominal bleeding. The latter may make mechanical ventilation impossible until relieved. The prone position may reduce compliance by up to 50%.

KEYPOINT

Compliance is a fundamental property of the respiratory system, which, although difficult to measure, determines the important lung volume properties.

TECHNIQUE: MEASUREMENT OF STATIC COMPLIANCE *IN VIVO*

To measure the compliance of the lung alone *in vivo*, transpulmonary (transmural pressure) must be determined across a range of volumes. The transpulmonary pressure is defined as the pressure difference between the alveoli and pleural cavity. For static conditions to apply, the measurements must be performed during breath-holding.

Pleural pressure is approximated by oesophageal pressure, which may be measured with an oesophageal balloon transducer. As there is no airflow through the respiratory tract during breath-holding, alveolar pressure is equal to pressure at the airway opening. Volume changes may be measured by spirometry.

Combined respiratory system compliance is easier to measure under anaesthesia as it requires muscle relaxation. The inflation pressure measured is the difference between alveolar and ambient pressure, rather than alveolar and pleural as in lung compliance. Intensive care unit ventilators calculate combined compliance automatically.

TYPICAL VALUES

Chest wall compliance	200 ml/cm H_2O inflation pressure (2 l/kPa)
Lung compliance	150 ml/cm H_2O (1.5 l/kPa)
Combined compliance	85 ml/cm H_2O (0.85 l/kPa)

NB Greater pressures than these are needed to inflate the chest, due to additional *airway resistance* (see Chapter 9).

Compliance is a reciprocal quantity (i.e. inversely proportional to the recoil), so that the combined compliance is *less* that the sum of its components.

$$\text{Total recoil} = \text{chest wall recoil} + \text{lung recoil}$$

or

$$\frac{1}{\text{combined compliance}} = \frac{1}{\text{chest wall compliance}} + \frac{1}{\text{lung compliance}}$$

CLINICAL ASPECTS OF COMPLIANCE

Patients with reduced compliance tend to breathe rapidly with very small breaths. Emphysema is the only cause of increased compliance. In this condition, the lack of elastic recoil causes airway collapse in exhalation and the expiratory phase of breathing is prolonged.

Summary

- Compliance is a measure of the distensibility of the lung and chest wall.
- Reduced lung compliance is a feature of interstitial lung disease, pulmonary oedema and ARDS (i.e. the lungs are stiffer).
- Increased lung compliance is seen only in emphysema.

6

LUNG VOLUMES

Key definitions

- TLC Total lung capacity
- V_A Alveolar volume
- RV Residual volume
- FRC Functional residual capacity
- V_T Tidal volume
- CV Closing volume

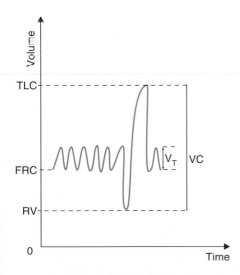

Fig. 6.1

Lung volumes

This spirometer trace is from a normal subject. The subject takes six normal breaths, then breathes all the way out to RV, and then all the way in to TLC, and then resumes normal tidal breathing. Lung volume automatically returns to the same FRC at the end of each normal tidal breath.

TLC, total lung capacity; FRC, functional residual capacity; RV, residual volume; V_T, tidal volume; VC, vital capacity.

TOTAL LUNG CAPACITY

This is the volume of gas in the lungs at the end of a maximal inspiration.

Physiology

As the lung expands, it becomes stiffer at higher volumes. In inspiration, the lung reaches TLC when the force generated by the respiratory muscles balances the recoil of the lungs.

- A reduction in TLC defines a restrictive defect.
- TLC is often increased in obstructive disorders. In emphysema, the increased pulmonary compliance allows the inspiratory muscles to distend the lung to greater volumes than normal. TLC may be transiently increased during an asthma attack, returning to normal at an interval of up to several weeks later.

Causes of reduced TLC (see Tables 2.1–2.3).

Technique

TLC cannot be measured using spirometry, as it is not possible to exhale the entire contents of the lung. There are two methods of measurement:

1. Multiple breath helium dilution

The subject breathes through tubing, which is then switched into a closed ventilatory system containing an air/helium mix. The helium concentration falls as the volume of gas in the system equilibrates with that in the lungs. After 5–10 minutes, when mixing is complete, the lung volume is calculated from the ratio of the starting concentration of helium to the equilibration value. The volume measured is the lung capacity when the subject was first switched into the circuit, which is usually performed at FRC.

A maximal inspiration is then taken, and TLC is the sum of the FRC and the measured volume inspired. This technique tends to underestimate TLC in emphysema, as little helium enters underventilated bullae during the period of equilibration (Fig. 6.2).

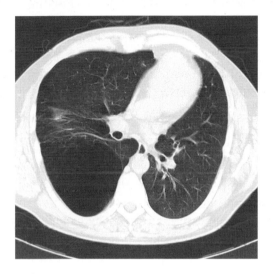

Fig. 6.2

CT scan of a patient with bullous emphysema

As can be seen, there is a large bulla in the dorsal region of the right lung. If this is ventilated by a communication with the bronchial tree, it forms a large pool of dead space. Ventilation of bullae may be assessed by performing CT scans in inspiration and expiration to assess change in size relative to the cross-sectional area of the thorax. Bullae may exert compression on surrounding parenchyma, as evidenced here by distortion of the overlying vasculature. Surgical resection ('bullectomy') is often helpful.

2. Whole-body plethysmography

This produces a more accurate value, but may slightly overestimate TLC.

Typical value

TLC is approximately 6 l in an adult, with a 53% contribution from the right lung, and 47% from the left.

ALVEOLAR VOLUME (TLC − V_D)

There is confusion around usage of the term 'alveolar volume'. To physiologists, it means the part of the breath that reaches the alveoli, i.e. tidal volume minus anatomical dead space – see the alveolar ventilation equation (Chapter 10) and the Bohr equation (Chapter 12). For the purposes of lung transfer factor calculation, however, it is necessary to make a measurement of the lung volume into which carbon monoxide diffuses during the technique. This is TLC minus dead space, and is also given the name 'alveolar volume'. The following paragraphs refer to this latter 'alveolar volume'.

The alveolar volume is measured routinely by single breath helium dilution, as a necessary part of measurement of TL_{CO}.

Technique: single breath helium dilution

The volume into which helium equilibrates during a 10-second breath-hold at full inspiration is equal to the alveolar volume plus that of the conducting airways. The conducting airway volume is 150 ml ± body weight correction factor, and may be subtracted from the volume measured to give V_A.

Interpretation of V_A

In the presence of obstructive airways disease, the V_A measurement is rather lower than TLC measured by the multiple-breath helium dilution method above, as the air/helium mixture does not equilibrate throughout obstructed segments during the single breath-hold manoeuvre. This TLC–V_A disparity or 'volume gap' is a useful index of the extent of air-trapping occurring in airways disease and emphysema.

RESIDUAL VOLUME

This is the volume of gas remaining in the lungs at the end of a maximal expiration.

Physiology

In a young subject, expiration can go no further when the ribs are apposed. With increasing age, lung elasticity is lost and airways collapse in extreme exhalation, causing air-trapping, which limits expiration to higher residual volumes. As a result, the RV rises from 25% of TLC at age 20, to 40% at age 70. Residual volume is normally expressed as a proportion of TLC.

● TLC is the sum of vital capacity and residual volume.

Causes of increased residual volume
Airways disease

An increase in RV is a cardinal abnormality of airway disease, caused by air-trapping in units that do not empty in expiration. Air-trapping may be seen radiologically in high-resolution computed tomography (CT) cuts of the lungs taken in expiration (Fig. 6.3). Despite the increased TLC, which may be seen in emphysema, the increase in RV is invariably greater, so that vital capacity is below normal.

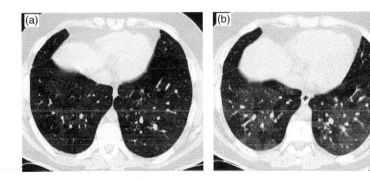

Fig. 6.3

Air-trapping

The two CT scans are of the same patient in inspiration (a) and in expiration (b). Both show a 'mosaic' pattern, more marked in expiration (b). The blacker regions of (b) have failed to empty of air in the normal way. The lighter regions are the more normal lung that has emptied of air. This illustrates air-trapping. This patient had airways disease caused by obliterative bronchiolitis.

The secondary pulmonary lobule may be defined as the smallest lung unit marginated by connective tissue septae, and usually comprises around 12 acini. An acinus is the portion of lung supplied by a first order respiratory bronchiole.

- If the RV is not increased in a subject with airway obstruction, it may be an indication of a coexisting restrictive disorder.

Expiratory muscle weakness

In respiratory muscle weakness, there is usually involvement of both inspiratory and expiratory groups, with isolated diaphragmatic palsy being an exception. Weakness of *expiratory* muscles reduces the force that can be applied to expelling air from the thorax. The characteristic pattern of any muscle weakness is a reduced TLC with an increased RV. The maximum expiratory flow volume curve shows a prolonged tail as the patient is no longer able to sustain a forceful expiration.

Chronic left ventricular failure

Chronic pulmonary venous congestion causes an increase in the residual volume of the lung by up to 40%. The vascular and interstitial congestion make the lung poorly compressible by the chest wall.

KEYPOINT

RV is usually normal with restrictive pulmonary disease.

FUNCTIONAL RESIDUAL CAPACITY

FRC is the volume of gas remaining in the lungs at the end of a normal relaxed expiration.

Physiology

Relaxation volume (V_r) is the volume at which the tendency for the lung to collapse is balanced by the tendency of the chest wall to expand, with the muscles in a neutral state. This is the natural endpoint of a relaxed tidal expiration, i.e. functional residual capacity.

If the lung is separated from the chest wall, as at thoracotomy, it collapses to a minimum volume (MV), determined by its elasticity. This is less than residual volume and normally about 10% of TLC. The separated chest wall expands to approximately FRC +1 l. The FRC of the combined system is between these two points.

The FRC forms a reservoir of oxygen. In the event of sudden loss of consciousness with apnoea, oxygen transfer continues from the air remaining in the residual capacity. This maintains oxygen saturation for approximately 1 minute. If there were no air left in the lung at the end of expiration, desaturation would occur instantly, even on normal exhalation.

If a subject breathes 100% oxygen before losing consciousness (as in the induction of anaesthesia), saturation is maintained for much longer, owing to the fivefold greater oxygen concentration in the FRC.

Typical value

FRC normally occurs at 50% of total lung capacity and may increase slightly with age, owing to reduced recoil and elasticity.

Resting tidal volume is normally about 500 ml. In mechanical ventilation, approximately 7–10 ml/kg is usually used.

Factors affecting FRC
Physiological factors

Exertion
In relaxed tidal breathing, expiration is a passive process during which the expiratory muscles are relaxed. With increasing demand for ventilation, as in exercise, the expiratory muscles are engaged. Functional residual capacity then reduces toward RV.

Posture
FRC decreases by 25% (mean reduction from 3.0 to 2.2 l) when supine, owing to extra loading of the diaphragm by the weight of the abdominal viscera.

Anaesthesia

Induction of anaesthesia brings about a further reduction in FRC of 15–20% below the reduction seen in the supine subject. The reduction is seen whether neuromuscular blockade is used or not, and occurs with all anaesthetic drugs. This reduces FRC to around the level of the closing capacity.

Pathological factors

Fibrotic lung disease

The lungs are smaller and stiffer, and the FRC is smaller.

Obstructive airway disease

FRC is increased in emphysema owing to air-trapping and lower recoil (greater compliance) of the lung.

Obesity

Obesity causes a marked reduction in FRC.

Clinical aspects of FRC: PEEP and CPAP

Mechanical ventilation works by providing positive airway pressure to inflate the lung. This is in contrast to the spontaneously breathing subject whose respiratory muscles inflate the lungs by transmission of negative pressure from the pleura to the airways. Expiration in both cases is effected passively by development of positive pressure in the airways, transmitted from the passive recoil of the chest wall and lungs. The subject undergoing mechanical ventilation, therefore, has positive airway pressure throughout the respiratory cycle.

Positive end-expiratory pressure (PEEP) is applied to patients with acute respiratory failure undergoing mechanical ventilation. It is a small pressure applied to the airway during expiration, against which a subject must breathe to exhale. This has the favourable effect of increasing FRC. If all other ventilatory parameters remained the same, the tidal volume would, therefore, be reduced, as inspiration would start at a higher volume and end at the same volume. To maintain the tidal volume in the mechanically ventilated patient, the inspiratory pressure is also increased to raise inspiratory volume by a similar amount.

PEEP could theoretically be applied to spontaneously breathing patients, but limiting it to expiration would necessitate use of a valve that switched to air at ambient pressure on inspiration. To maintain the same tidal volume, a spontaneously breathing patient would then have to raise inspiratory volume by their own effort, thereby increasing the work of breathing. Pure PEEP is never used alone in those breathing spontaneously.

Spontaneously breathing patients may benefit from the effects of PEEP but it is more beneficial to apply it throughout the respiratory cycle. When using this continuous positive airways pressure (CPAP), expiration ends with positive airway pressure, as in PEEP. Inspiration, however, also starts with positive airway pressure and, when added to the negative pleural pressure of inspiration, this achieves a greater end-inspiratory volume without increasing the subject's work of breathing. CPAP, therefore, aids inspiration, whilst providing a resistance to expiration. CPAP may be provided to spontaneously breathing patients through a tightly fitting face mask, which creates a seal around the nose and mouth.

The effect of both PEEP and CPAP is to increase FRC. In normal subjects, such as those undergoing mechanical ventilation during elective surgery, this is of little benefit. However, in patients with respiratory failure, it has several favourable effects:

1 The increase in FRC relative to closing capacity increases the amount of lung that is aerated throughout the respiratory cycle, improving $\dot{V}/\dot{Q}$ matching and oxygenation (see 'Closing capacity').
2 Consolidated lung tends to collapse at low volumes and the elevation of FRC recruits such segments to active ventilation, improving oxygenation.
3 In patients with pulmonary oedema, increasing the volume of aerated lung increases the capacity of the pulmonary interstitium for water and reduces the volume of alveolar oedema.

4   In patients with stiff and poorly compliant lungs, the increase in FRC shifts the lung to a more favourable point on the pressure/volume curve, so that less work is done by the subject to inflate the lung in inspiration.

5   In spontaneously breathing patients, face-mask CPAP is used to treat obstructive sleep apnoea (OSA). In OSA, the pharynx tends to collapse under the negative pressure of inspiration whilst asleep; it accompanies severe snoring. By raising airway pressure, the upper airway is splinted open during inspiration.

Technique of FRC measurement

FRC is measured by helium dilution. It is a crucial physiological parameter but not generally used to characterize respiratory disease.

CLOSING CAPACITY

● Closing capacity
● Closing volume (equals closing capacity − RV)

In expiration, as lung volume falls, a point is reached where airways in the basal segments of the lung close and become airless. The lung volume at which this occurs is the closing capacity. The pulmonary blood flow reaching this zone is perfusing non-ventilated lung. Pulmonary venous blood, therefore, returns to the left heart less than fully saturated and there is consequently a reduction in arterial Po_2.

Factors affecting closing capacity

Age

In the young subject, the closing capacity is little more than residual volume, and so all airways are permanently open, except in extreme expiration (Fig. 6.4) However, there is a significant increase in closing capacity with age, so that, by the fifth decade, it is equal to FRC in the supine position, and by the seventh, equal to FRC standing. If closing capacity is

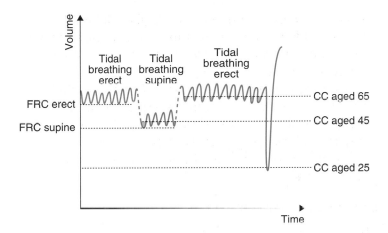

Fig. 6.4

Closure of dependent airways during tidal breathing

The trace is of a subject taking tidal respirations in the standing and supine positions. FRC is lower when supine. As lung volume falls during expiration, a point comes when airways in the dependent parts of the lung start to close. This volume is called the closing capacity. The closing volume is the difference between closing capacity and RV.

At age 25, closing capacity (CC) is very low, so that dependent airways are closed only in extreme expiration, when lung volume is close to residual volume.

By age 45, the closing capacity increases, so that airways close during normal tidal respiration in the supine position. (The shaded area shows the portion of the respiratory cycle during which airways are closed.)

By 65, closing capacity has increased to above FRC in the standing position.

above FRC, dependent airways will be closed for some part of each respiratory cycle. (FRC changes little with age.)

Posture

As FRC is less when supine, tidal breathing more closely approaches the closing capacity in this position. When measured supine, closing capacity is equal to the FRC by the age of 45. As FRC decreases further under anaesthesia, there it causes a further reduction in oxygenation.

KEYPOINT

The increase in closing capacity with age is thought to be the mechanism of the reduction in 'normal' arterial Po_2 with age, from 13.3 kPa at age 20, to 10.6 kPa at age 70.

Measurement of closing volume

Closing volume is rarely measured, as it gives little diagnostic information about disease within the lung. It remains an important physiological entity, which explains the changes in arterial oxygenation seen in postural change, anaesthesia and ageing.

Summary

Lung volume measurement is a sensitive test which is often abnormal in lung disease before spirometry.

Typical disease patterns:

	TLC	RV	RV/TLC
Obstructive	↑	↑	↑
Restrictive lung disease	↓	↔	↑
Muscle weakness	↓	↑	↑

The most useful and sensitive volume indices are:

- Obstructive disease   an increase in RV /TLC
- Restrictive lung disease   a decrease in TLC, vital capacity

7

DIFFUSION CAPACITY

Key definitions

- TL_{CO} Transfer factor of the lung for carbon monoxide
  This is the total diffusing capacity of the lung for carbon monoxide (syn. DL_{CO} = Diffusion capacity of the lung for carbon monoxide)
- K_{CO} Transfer coefficient
  Diffusing capacity of the lung per unit lung volume. This measure is standardized for the alveolar volume.

Physiology: diffusive conductance

TL_{CO} describes the total diffusing capacity of the lung for carbon monoxide. Physically it represents the diffusive conductance (ease of transfer) of carbon monoxide across the blood gas barrier. It is a measure of the surface area available for gas transfer, and the integrity of that surface. As a function of both alveolar volume and diffusion efficiency, it is affected by alterations in either.

To standardize the measurement to a subject's lung volume, the parameter K_{CO} is used:

$$TL_{CO} = K_{CO} \times V_A$$

where V_A = alveolar volume[1]
       = total lung capacity − anatomical dead space

K_{CO} is a measure of the diffusive conductance per unit alveolar volume.

---

[1]See 'Alveolar volume' in Chapter 6 for the meaning of this term

---

KEYPOINTS

- TL_{CO} and K_{CO} are measures of the gas-exchanging capacity of the lung. They are sensitive indices of the integrity of the blood-gas interface.
- As a function of both alveolar volume and diffusion capacity, TL_{CO} is affected by alterations in either.

K_{CO} VERSUS TL_{CO}: INTERPRETATION

If a proportion of the lung volume is removed, the surface area available for gas exchange is reduced. The composite function TL_{CO} is, therefore, reduced according to the proportion of volume lost. Assuming cardiac output remains unchanged, however, and the remaining lung tissue is functionally good, then increased perfusion improves carbon monoxide transfer. The volume-standardized measure K_{CO} is, therefore, increased by loss of volume. Surgical resection is the only true example of this kind as it leaves normal lung tissue. Following pneumonectomy, there is a reduction in TL_{CO} with an increase in K_{CO} by up to 150%.

In a similar way, a disease may obliterate alveoli scattered throughout both lungs, but leave other units unaffected (Fig. 7.1).

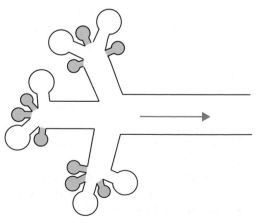

Fig. 7.1

Interstitial lung disease
Patchy obliteration of alveolar units causing loss of lung volume. This patient may have a preserved K_{CO}, but will undoubtedley have reduction in V_A and TL_{CO}.

The V_A and, therefore, TL_{CO} are reduced. *If the function of remaining units is intact,* then the increased perfusion of remaining units increases the volume-standardized measure K_{CO}. Invariably, however, any disease process causes *some* impairment of remaining alveoli, so that, at best, K_{CO} tends to be normal or slightly increased. A more typical pattern is therefore reduction of TL_{CO} with preservation of K_{CO}. This is classically the case in sarcoid.

On the other hand, alveoli may be obliterated by a disease process, which also significantly impairs the remaining alveoli. Pulmonary oedema is such an example. If alveoli are flooded by pulmonary oedema, there is a reduction in V_A and, therefore, TL_{CO}. The presence of interstitial oedema, however, impairs remaining units, so gas transfer is also reduced when standardized for V_A, giving a low K_{CO}.

This discussion is expanded in 'Causes of reduced TL_{CO}'. It is detailed further in the text by Hughes and Pride (see Bibliography), whose work has contributed much to this area.

CAUSES OF REDUCED TL$_{CO}$

1 Reduced alveolar volume (V$_A$)
Discrete loss of alveolar units
This is where alveolar volume is lost but the remaining tissue functions normally. After pneumonectomy, K_{CO} may increase to 150% of predicted, although TL_{CO} is reduced. Pulmonary collapse, local destruction of a segment post pneumonia or TB, may have a similar effect.

The same term is applied to disease that obliterates some alveoli, but leaves unaffected units working well. This is seen classically in sarcoid and may occur in the cellular variant of non-specific interstitial pneumonitis. It is likely, however, that any disease process that obliterates some alveoli will affect those remaining somewhat. Under these circumstances there is relative preservation of K_{CO} despite reduction of TL_{CO}.

Diffuse loss of alveolar units

This pattern is typified by most interstitial disease processes, which remove volume by obliteration of some alveoli but diffusely damage those remaining. TL_{CO} and K_{CO} are therefore both reduced.

Incomplete lung expansion

This is seen when chest wall or pleural disease restricts lung inflation. A pattern similar to that in discrete loss of alveolar units is seen. Where V_A is reduced by restriction of expansion, however, without loss of tissue *per se*, the unexpanded lung takes the form of a concertina that still presents a large surface for gas exchange. Although the TL_{CO} is, therefore, slightly reduced, the volume-specific measure K_{CO} may be increased greatly, by up to 200% predicted or more.

Airflow obstruction

As discussed under 'Alveolar volume' in Chapter 6, in airway obstruction the single breath measurement technique results in a low measurement of V_A, which is rather less than would be recorded by multiple-breath dilution as used for measurement of TLC. TL_{CO} is, therefore, reduced in proportion to the reduction of the measured V_A, with relative preservation of K_{CO}.

2 Reduction of K_{CO}

As a measure that is standardized to alveolar volume, K_{CO} primarily reflects the integrity of the pulmonary vasculature. Most lung diseases deleteriously affect K_{CO} (see Table 7.1 for a list of examples, which is not exhaustive).

CAUSES OF A RAISED K_{CO}

As discussed, the increased perfusion caused by loss of lung volume may increase K_{CO}, if the remaining tissue is normal.

Table 7.1 Causes of reduction of K_{CO}

Condition	Examples	Comment
Interstitial lung disease	Cryptogenic fibrosing alveolitis (CFA) Autoimmune Pneumoconioses Extrinsic allergic alveolitis (EAA)	K_{CO} often relatively preserved in sarcoid
Pulmonary vascular disease	Primary pulmonary hypertension Hepatopulmonary syndrome Pulmonary vasculitis Pulmonary arteriovenous malformations	TL_{CO} and K_{CO} often relatively preserved in pulmonary embolism* K_{CO} may be raised in vasculitis in the presence of fresh haemorrhage
Cardiac	Persistent pulmonary venous hypertension Pulmonary oedema Eisenmenger syndrome	
Airways disease	Emphysema Bronchiolitis Bronchiectasis	K_{CO} and TL_{CO} normal or high in asthma

*This is believed to be due to perfusion of the pulmonary circulation distal to the emboli by blood from the bronchial circulation entering the pulmonary circulation through anastomoses. This bronchial artery blood also binds and transports carbon monoxide.

K_{CO} is also raised when perfusion is increased due to left to right shunt or any cause of high cardiac output, such as anaemia.

Alveolar haemorrhage also increases K_{CO} due to the binding of CO by fresh blood in the alveolar space. The effect is dependent upon patency of the airways supplying the areas of haemorrhage. This may be seen in the pulmonary vasculitides, such as Goodpasture's, Wegener's and systemic lupus erythematosus (SLE); the same phenomenon occurs in idiopathic pulmonary haemosiderosis.

Summary

- TL_{CO} is a sensitive test, which may be abnormal in lung disease before other tests are deranged.
- TL_{CO} is used particularly to follow the course of diffuse lung disease.
- K_{CO} is needed to interpret the diffusion capacity where there is coexisting reduction of lung volume.
- K_{CO} is raised where there is discrete loss of alveolar volume, high cardiac output or pulmonary haemorrhage.

8

RESPIRATORY MUSCLE POWER

Skeletal muscle disease often involves the respiratory muscles and commonly causes respiratory impairment (Table 8.1). Occasionally muscle disease presents dramatically with acute respiratory failure, which invariably causes diagnostic confusion. Since the advent of non-invasive ventilation, there is an increasing population of patients with respiratory failure due to severe respiratory muscle disease who are now maintained by this means.

Table 8.1 Neuromuscular causes of respiratory failure

Conditions	Examples
Central nervous system disease	Motor neurone disease*
	Poliomyelitis
	Cervical cord injury
Neuropathies	Guillain–Barré
	Bilateral diaphragmatic paralysis*
	Critical illness neuropathy
Neuromuscular junction disorder	Myasthenia gravis
	Botulism
Muscle disease	Polymyositis
	Dystrophies (Duchenne, spinal muscular atrophy and limb-girdle dystrophy)
	Myopathies especially acid maltase deficiency*, mitochondrial myopathy

* Respiratory failure may be the presenting complaint.

INVESTIGATION OF RESPIRATORY MUSCLE STRENGTH

This often takes the form of a progression of tests, each with increasing specificity to exclude the diagnosis of respiratory muscle weakness.

Vital capacity

VC is a useful screening test. The sensitivity of the test may be increased by measurement supine, when the weight of the abdominal viscera applies additional load to the diaphragm. Normally the VC supine is within 5% of that erect. A disparity of greater than 25% between the erect and supine VC is definitely abnormal, and indicative of neuromuscular disease.

- A normal supine VC excludes clinically important respiratory muscle weakness.
- The typical defect seen in respiratory muscle weakness is reduction of TLC and FVC with an increased RV. The effect on FRC is variable. (In restrictive lung disease, RV tends to remain unchanged.)
- The K_{CO} may be dramatically increased to greater than 200% predicted in respiratory muscle weakness.
- The ability to cough requires good muscle power, and is crucial to clear secretions and prevent infection. If the vital capacity is less that 30 ml/kg, the ability to cough is likely to be impaired.

Clinical aspects of muscle weakness
Acute neuromuscular failure

Guillain–Barré syndrome is the commonest cause of this presentation and is life-threatening, although patients usually make a full recovery. It requires expert management.

Vital capacity is the best means of monitoring the progression of respiratory muscle impairment in this condition. Peak flow is not particularly helpful. A vital capacity of at least 15 ml/kg is required to maintain spontaneous ventilation, and a drop to less than this is an indication for intubation and mechanical ventilation.

Ventilation should be considered earlier if the patient is tiring or there is pharyngeal incoordination so that the airway is poorly protected.

PITFALL

In acute neuromuscular failure, blood gases may not be abnormal until respiratory arrest is absolutely imminent, and should *not* be relied upon to assess the patient.

Myasthenia gravis is a chronic disease of the neuromuscular transmission, in which patients are prone to crises with acute respiratory failure. The vital capacity is of less use in predicting respiratory failure during crises in this condition, as the course is more fluctuating.

Chronic neuromuscular disease
● In chronic respiratory muscle disease, a VC of less than one-third of normal has been found to predict impending respiratory failure.
● Arterial Pco_2 rises gradually in chronic respiratory muscle disease. Decompensated respiratory failure may follow soon after elevation of Pco_2 above normality.

Because of the extra load placed on the diaphragm when supine, and the effects of sleep on respiratory control, arterial Pco_2 tends to rise overnight in patients with muscle weakness. Patients with neuromuscular disease may complain of morning headaches caused by nocturnal carbon dioxide retention.

Mouth pressures

- MIP   Maximum inspiratory pressure
- MEP   Maximum expiratory pressure

These measurements may be useful in the presence of equivocal supine VC manoeuvre. Maximum inspiratory pressure is the more useful measure, as the inspiratory muscles play the more important role in breathing. It is measured at FRC or RV.

Normal MIP is approximately 120 cm H_2O. A value of >80 cm H_2O excludes clinically important disease. A MIP of <30% normal predicts impending respiratory failure. A MIP of less than 30 cm H_2O in a ventilated patient is associated with failure to wean.

Maximum expiratory pressure is measured at TLC. Although less useful in predicting the ability to breathe, it gives information about the subject's ability to cough. A weak cough is an important feature of decline in muscle power, as it impairs ability to clear airway secretions and predisposes to pneumonia.

Portable hand-held meters may be used in the clinic or at the bedside, and are adequate for making routine mouth pressure measurements, although more accurate measurements can be made in the laboratory.

Transdiaphragmatic measurements

- Sniff P_{DI} Difference between gastric and oesophageal pressures, simultaneously measured by catheter placement.

This is the most reproducible and accurate volitional test of inspiratory muscle strength, although it is not widely available. It may be indicated if equivocal results are obtained by less invasive tests. Catheter-mounted balloon transducers are placed into the oesophagus and stomach via the nasal route. The subject is asked to take a hard sniff, and the transdiaphragmatic pressure is the difference between that measured in the stomach and the oesophagus. The procedure is surprisingly well tolerated, if performed expertly.

● Twitch P_{DI} Difference between gastric and oesophageal pressures, simultaneously measured by catheter placement during magnetic stimulation of the phrenic nerves.

The twitch P_{DI} also measures transdiaphragmatic pressure but, instead of performing measurement during a sniff, magnetic stimulation is painlessly applied to the phrenic nerves in the cervical region.

This provides the gold standard measurement of inspiratory muscle strength and is useful in assessment of complex problems, e.g. in connective tissue disease where there may be pulmonary fibrosis reducing lung volumes and associated myopathy. It may also be helpful in assessing breathlessness in patients with equivocal results from other tests of muscle strength.

Radiological assessment of muscle strength

If the diaphragm is paralysed, it moves paradoxically in respiration, being sucked upward into the thorax in inspiration. This may be visualized by fluoroscopy or ultrasound.

However, many patients with diaphragmatic paralysis learn to contract the abdominal muscles during expiration, displacing the diaphragm cranially. At the start of inspiration, the abdominals are relaxed, allowing passive descent of the diaphragm, which may give a misleading radiological picture. This makes this means of assessment rather insensitive.

Summary

Respiratory failure may complicate generalized muscle weakness, and may be the first presentation of the condition. A normal supine vital capacity excludes clinically important disease. In equivocal cases, more information may be gained by mouth pressure measurements. The gold standard test is transdiaphragmatic pressure, which is best measured during magnetic stimulation of the diaphragm. Radiological assessment of diaphragmatic weakness is insensitive.

9

AIRWAY RESISTANCE

Key definitions

- R_{aw} Airway resistance
- G_{aw} Airway conductance
- sGaw   Specific airway conductance

(pronounced 'raw', 'gore' and 's-gore', respectively.)

Physiology: airway resistance

The force needed by the inspiratory muscles to inflate the lungs is greater than the elastic recoil alone. This additional impedance is airway resistance, which originates from friction between air and mucosa. Work done against these resistive forces is lost by dissipation as heat.

Airway resistance creates a pressure difference between the mouth and the alveoli. Under conditions of laminar flow, the airway resistance is analogous to electrical resistance in an Ohmic conductor, and defined by the equation:

$$\text{Resistance} = \frac{\text{Pressure difference}}{\text{Flow rate}}$$

The following equation derived from the Poiseuille equation describes the factors that influence resistance in a parallel-sided tube under conditions of laminar flow:

$$R = \frac{8 \times \text{length} \times \text{viscosity}}{\pi \times \text{radius}^4}$$

Airflow in the upper airways, however, is mainly turbulent. Under these circumstances, resistance to flow is greater than would be predicted by the Poiseuille equation. Resistance to turbulent flow is proportional to the density of the inspired gas and the square of the flow rate, and inversely proportional to the fifth power of airway radius. The resistance to turbulent flow is independent of the gas viscosity.

KEYPOINTS

The total impedance to airflow comprises:

- An elastic component, due to the recoil of the lung parenchyma and chest wall.
- A resistive component, which originates from friction between air and airway.

FACTORS AFFECTING AIRWAY RESISTANCE

Physiological factors

Airway tone

Most normal subjects have some resting airway tone, mediated by the vagus nerve. This may be abolished by muscarinic antagonists or beta adrenoceptor agonists, resulting in a 30% reduction in airway resistance.

Lung volume

At smaller lung volumes, the airways are compressed to a narrower diameter, causing a reciprocal increase in resistance. Airway resistance is, therefore, a function of the volume at which it is measured. The value may be standardized by measurement at FRC.

Flow-related airway collapse

Physiology: forced expiratory flows

In relaxed tidal breathing, pleural pressure remains negative throughout the respiratory cycle, owing to the different relaxation volumes of the lung and chest wall. During a forced expiration, however, the expiratory muscles are actively contracting to expel air from the thorax. This generates positive intrapleural pressure.

Therefore, during a forced expiration from TLC, two forces are active in expelling air from the lung:

1 The elastic recoil of the respiratory system, seeking to return the lung to FRC.
2 Positive intrapleural pressure generated by the respiratory muscles.

However, as the thoracic cage squeezes alveoli, forcing air out, it also compresses airways. This creates a tendency for airway collapse, especially late in expiration. Therefore, the same intrapleural pressure that is *driving* expiration is also *obstructing* it, so the forces tend to cancel out (Fig. 4.10; see p. 32). The elastic recoil of the tissue in which the airways are embedded is important in maintaining their patency.

KEYPOINT

Airway collapse is the rate-limiting factor that determines maximum flows during a maximal expiratory effort. The tendency to collapse is governed by the lung's properties of parenchymal elasticity (where recoil originates) and airway resistance. FEV_1 is determined principally by these parameters, rather than the amount of effort applied, making it reproducible. Peak flow occurs earlier in expiration, before airway collapse occurs, and is more effort dependent.

Pathological factors
Airway obstruction
By reducing the airway calibre, secretions, foreign body, tumour or extrinsic compression may increase resistance to the point that the work of breathing is not sustainable.

Asthma
A diurnal variation in airway tone is seen in normal subjects, with a peak at around 4.00 am. In asthma there is a state of increased airway reactivity, which may cause life-threatening bronchospasm. Additional airway obstruction may be caused by mucus plugs produced by associated airway inflammation, and are a frequent post-mortem finding in patients who have died of acute asthma.

Clinical aspects of airflow
Use of helium to reduce airways resistance
Under conditions of turbulent flow, resistance may be greatly reduced by breathing oxygen mixed with helium rather than nitrogen. The airways present less resistance to this molecule under conditions of turbulent flow, owing to its lower density. This may occasionally be useful as a palliative measure in airflow obstruction, where turbulent flow is encountered.

Airway resistance in the mechanically ventilated patient
When expanding the lungs and chest wall with positive pressure ventilation, three sources of impedance are met:

- static compliance of the chest wall
- static compliance of the lung
- airway resistance.

Very approximately, for a 700 ml breath, given over an inspiratory period of 1 sec, an airway pressure of 15 cm H_2O will be required. About 5 cm H_2O is required to overcome each of the above components.

Technique for measurement of airway resistance

The subject takes tidal breaths in a body plethysmograph. The air breathed is drawn from and discharged into the plethysmograph chamber. There is, therefore, no net change in the volume of gas in the chamber throughout the respiratory cycle. Small measurable changes in air pressure during the respiratory cycle result from compression and rarefaction of alveolar gas; from these, airway resistance may be calculated.

R_{aw} has a hyperbolic relationship to lung volume, rising sharply below FRC. Its reciprocal, conductance (G_{aw}), therefore, has a straight-line relationship to volume. The specific conductance (sG_{aw}) is a volume-independent measure of resistance/conductance, which may be derived graphically.

Normal values

Airway resistance (R_{aw})   1.5–2 cm H_2O.s/l
                                  (measured at FRC)
Specific conductance (sG_{aw})   0.13–0.35 cm H_2O/s

Clinical aspects of airway resistance

- Airway resistance measurement gives greater sensitivity in assessing response to bronchial provocation than does FEV_1.

KEYPOINT

When mechanically ventilating the lungs against high airway resistance, high inflation pressures are needed. These pressures are not transmitted to the alveoli but fall down a continuous pressure gradient along the length of the conducting pathway. The alveoli, therefore, may experience normal pressures.

The situation is different when ventilating stiff lungs with reduced compliance. High airway pressures are also needed, but the increased stiffness lies in the tissues, and not the airways. Greater airway pressure is, therefore, transmitted to the alveoli.

This accuracy also has applications for studies of airway pharmacology.

● Airway resistance measurement may be useful to assess airways disease in the subject who cannot perform a forced expiratory manoeuvre, owing to coughing or subject compliance.

Airway resistance is truly independent of effort, and is not subject to a patient's volition.

Summary

Airway resistance is a fundamental property of the lungs that determines flow. Resistance is inversely proportional to the fourth power of airway radius, so that halving the diameter causes a 16-fold increase in resistance, or greater under conditions of turbulent flow.

Resistance is not commonly measured, however, as spirometry and peak flow measurements give broadly the same information.

PART

II

BLOOD GAS INTERPRETATION

Key definitions
- P_aO_2 Tension of oxygen in arterial blood
- P_aCO_2 Tension of carbon dioxide in arterial blood

Physiology: concentrations of gases in liquids

Arterial PO_2 and PCO_2 are the tensions of the gases in blood. Henry's law states that the concentration (c) of gas (x) dissolved in a solution is equal to the product of its partial pressure at the surface and its solubility coefficient (α):

$$c = \alpha\, P_x$$

If a liquid is in equilibrium with the gas at its surface, the partial pressure of a gas at the surface is the same as the tension of the gas in physical solution in the liquid. (Tension is synonymous with partial pressure and is applied particularly to gases dissolved in a liquid, whereas partial pressure tends to be used for gases in gas.)

As CO_2 is carried in physical solution, the arterial PCO_2 provides a measurement of the CO_2 content of a volume of blood. Most oxygen, however, is chemically bound to haemoglobin and, although this is in equilibrium with oxygen in physical solution,

P_{O_2} directly measures only the latter. Haemoglobin saturation must be measured to quantify the volume of oxygen in whole blood (see 'Oxygen content' in Chapter 13).

Introduction to blood gas interpretation

Arterial P_{CO_2} gives information about ventilation, whereas P_{O_2} gives information about the efficiency of gas exchange. Arterial P_{CO_2} should be examined in conjunction with pH, followed by arterial P_{O_2} with haemoglobin saturation S_aO_2. Each of these parameters is covered in its own chapter.

Respiratory failure

Respiratory failure exists when arterial P_{O_2} is less than 8 kPa. Knowledge of the arterial P_{CO_2} allows classification by pathophysiology:

Type 1 (hypoxic)   Arterial P_{CO_2} – normal or low
Type 2 (hypercapnic) Arterial P_{CO_2} – high (>7 kPa)

Type 2 failure is *ventilatory* failure, i.e. there is inadequate air *reaching* the gas-exchanging area. This may be due to reduced ventilation or increased dead space.

In pure hypoxic (type 1) respiratory failure, sufficient oxygen reaches the alveoli, but ventilation is not well-matched with perfusion so that blood is shunted through underventilated alveolar units. This may occur regionally, e.g. through a collapsed lobe, or in units scattered throughout both lungs, e.g. in interstitial lung disease. The minute volume of ventilation is usually increased to compensate, and arterial P_{CO_2} is, therefore, low or normal.

KEYPOINT

Arterial P_{CO_2} primarily gives information about *ventilation*, whereas arterial P_{O_2} gives information about *efficiency of gas exchange*.

10

ASSESSMENT OF VENTILATION

ASSESSMENT OF ARTERIAL P_{CO_2}

Arterial P_{CO_2} quantifies *ventilation*. Its concentration in blood is determined by a number of factors:

Key definitions

- $\dot{V}_E$ Minute ventilation
  The total volume of air breathed in a minute. This is more conveniently measured (and therefore expressed) as the expired volume.
- $\dot{V}_A$ Alveolar ventilation
  The volume of air breathed in a minute, which reaches the gas-exchanging area.
- V_T Tidal volume
  The volume of air in each breath.
- V_D Dead space
  The volume of air in each breath that does not reach alveoli, where gas exchange is taking place.
- $\dot{V}_{CO2}$ Rate of CO_2 production.

Factors affecting arterial P_{CO_2}

Physiology: alveolar ventilation equation

Alveolar ventilation is the volume of air passing in and out of the alveoli each minute. Dead space (V_D) is the volume of inspired air that does not reach alveoli where gas exchange is taking place (see 'Dead space' in Chapter 12 for a fuller discussion). Therefore:

Alveolar ventilation = frequency of breathing × alveolar volume
= frequency of breathing × (tidal volume − dead space)

$$\dot{V}_A = f (V_T - V_D)$$

Alveolar ventilation is an important concept, as it is the primary determinant of alveolar CO_2 concentration, which in turn determines arterial P_{CO_2}. By considering CO_2 as a tracer substance, we can calculate alveolar ventilation as follows.

In the steady state, the quantity of CO_2 exhaled is equal to the quantity produced by the body and discharged into the alveoli. As alveolar CO_2 is continuously diluted into the volume of alveolar ventilation:

CO_2 production = alveolar CO_2 concentration × alveolar ventilation

Rearranging:

$$\text{Alveolar } CO_2 \text{ concentration} = \frac{CO_2 \text{ production}}{\text{alveolar ventilation}}$$

This is a form of the alveolar ventilation equation.

KEYPOINTS

- From the alveolar ventilation equation we see that alveolar concentration of CO_2 (and hence arterial P_{CO_2}) is proportional to the rate of production of CO_2 and inversely proportional to alveolar ventilation.
- In practice, a raised P_{CO_2} is invariably caused by underventilation, so that arterial P_{CO_2} is an index of ventilatory sufficiency. Only occasionally does increased production of CO_2 contribute. For causes, see Table 10.1.

- Arterial P_{CO_2} is not affected by impairment of diffusion across the blood–gas barrier.
- Whereas arterial P_{CO_2} depends primarily on the minute volume of ventilation, arterial P_{O_2} depends on the efficiency of ventilation/perfusion matching

Normal values of arterial P_{CO_2}

- At rest, alveolar ventilation is adjusted to maintain P_{CO_2} close to 5.3 kPa. It is not influenced by age. A P_{CO_2} of greater than 6.0 kPa is definitely abnormal.
- Because of the very large volume of CO_2 (around 120 l) held buffered in the body, it takes 20–30 minutes after a change in ventilation for a new steady state to be reached. In a situation of total respiratory arrest, P_{CO_2} rises by only about 0.4–0.8 kPa each minute. In contrast, total body oxygen content is much lower (around 1.5 l while breathing air), and P_{O_2} equilibrates within a minute or so.

CLINICAL ASPECTS OF ARTERIAL P_{CO_2}

Hypercapnia (high arterial P_{CO_2})

- A raised P_{CO_2} is usually significant as it is rarely above 6 kPa in healthy subjects.
- Many patients with chronic lung disease have a persistently-raised arterial P_{CO_2} of up to 8 kPa. If this is of long-standing, it is well tolerated and compensated; that is the pH is normal. P_{CO_2} must always be read in conjunction with pH.
- A patient becomes comatose when P_{CO_2} reaches 12–16 kPa.

Causes of hypercapnia
Hypoventilation
Underventilation of gas-exchanging alveoli is the commonest mechanism of hypercapnia. Dead space may be raised (for causes, see Table 12.1) and/or minute volume reduced (for causes, see Table 10.1).

Table 10.1 Causes of ventilatory failure

Condition	Comment
Airways disease	
COPD	Classically the 'blue bloater' subtype is hypercapnic, but arterial Pco_2 is also often raised in 'pink puffers'. Emphysematous destruction of alveoli results in dead space, but COPD patients also hypoventilate with a tolerance of hypercapnia which is poorly understood
Asthma	Rising Pco_2 is a sign of impending respiratory arrest
Upper airway obstruction	Reduction of luminal diameter may increase airway resistance to the point where minute ventilation cannot be maintained against the work of breathing. A raised Pco_2 in this context is a late sign and respiratory arrest may soon follow
Increased dead space	An increase in dead space reduces alveolar ventilation. This is normally compensated by an increased minute volume. However, if V_D/V_T is hugely increased (>0.65) ventilatory failure may result. This may be seen in ARDS or emphysema with large bullae communicating with the airway (see 'Dead space' in Chapter 12)
Chest wall disorder	
Pickwickian syndrome/ obesity hypoventilation syndrome	Gross obesity impairs movement of the thoracic wall, with resultant low minute volume. This is a common cause of a chronically raised Pco_2
Neuromuscular disease	Motor neurone disease, Guillain–Barré, bilateral diaphragmatic paralysis, muscular dystrophy, myopathy (see Chapter 8, 'Respiratory muscle power')
Reduced chest wall compliance	Pleural encasement (e.g. post-empyema), ankylosing spondylitis, thoracoplasty, scleroderma, circumferential burns
Loss of structural integrity	Flail chest
Central depression of respiratory drive	Severe hypoxaemia, brain lesion, drugs
Exhaustion	Any cause of acute respiratory distress, especially if associated with increased work of breathing, e.g. asthma, acute pulmonary oedema

Chronic obstructive pulmonary disease (COPD)
Certain conditions are characterized by a tendency to hypoventilate, and so retain CO_2. This is explicable in neuromuscular disorders, where the primary problem is in the chest wall, but less easily understood in COPD.

Some patients with COPD regulate their breathing so as to maintain a set arterial Po_2. They may tolerate an arterial Pco_2 that is chronically high but compensated, i.e. the pH is normal. This group forms a minority of COPD patients, which are usually called 'CO_2 retainers'. If supplementary oxygen is administered to CO_2 retainers, Pco_2 may rise in an uncontrolled manner.

When oxygen is given to CO_2 retainers during an acute exacerbation, it should initially be administered in a concentration of 24–28%, and blood gases checked after one hour. If the pH is satisfactory, the F_1O_2 may be increased until the Po_2 is greater than 7.6 kPa. Blood gases should be rechecked after any change in oxygen therapy[1].

The rise in Pco_2 brought about by uncontrolled supplementary oxygen may cause respiratory acidosis and progression to coma, i.e. CO_2 narcosis. Occasionally, in the worst cases of COPD, even 24% oxygen may be associated with a significant rise in Pco_2. Non-invasive ventilation may be helpful in such cases, by maintaining an adequate minute volume of ventilation.

PITFALL

The characteristic clinical signs of hypercapnia, i.e. venous dilatation, CO_2 retention flap (asterixis), papilloedema and confusion, are unreliable and frequently absent.

---

[1]BTS guidelines for the management of chronic obstructive pulmonary disease. The COPD Guidelines Group of the Standards of Care Committee of the BTS. Thorax 1997; 52 (Suppl 5): S1–28. Available at http://thorax.bmjjournals.com/cgi/reprint/52/suppl_5/S1.pdf.

> ## KEYPOINT
>
> Most patients who present acutely to hospital with diagnoses, such as asthma, pneumonia or pulmonary oedema, are in no danger of CO_2 retention. High-concentration oxygen is immediately life-saving and should never needlessly be withheld. The chronic COPD patient is usually recognizable from the history and examination.

Obesity hypoventilation syndrome (OHS)

This is a sleep apnoea syndrome usually occurring in the markedly obese, where there is nocturnal hypoventilation, caused by the combination of increased chest wall loading and upper airway obstruction during sleep. P_{CO_2} rises at night in normal subjects by around 0.5 kPa, but may rise to 12–13 kPa in OHS. The symptom of morning headache, caused by CO_2 retention overnight is characteristic. The diagnosis may be confirmed by sleep study with transcutaneous CO_2 monitoring. The treatment is nocturnal non-invasive ventilation.

Exhaustion

Arterial P_{CO_2} may rise in any patient with respiratory failure who becomes exhausted, and unable to maintain their ventilatory effort. This is particularly so in asthma, acute pulmonary oedema and upper airway obstruction, where the increased airways resistance or lung stiffness increases the work of breathing to an unsustainable level.

Patients in this situation are gravely ill. Lack of respiratory drive is not the problem and despite the high P_{CO_2}, high-concentration oxygen should be given, *while senior help is sought.* Brief apnoeas or a sudden reduction in respiratory rate are a sign of *imminent respiratory arrest.*

Increased production of CO_2

High production of CO_2 may contribute to a raised P_{CO_2}. This is uncommon but may occur in thyrotoxicosis, sepsis, malignant hyperthermia or rhabdomyolysis. For a clinically significant rise to occur, however, there is usually coexisting ventilatory failure.

In critically ill patients with ventilatory failure, CO_2 production may be reduced by use of feeds that minimize carbohydrate in favour of substrates that are metabolized with a lower respiratory quotient, i.e. lipid. This may be a useful manoeuvre when ventilatory function is extremely marginal.

Hypocapnia (low arterial P_{CO_2})
Causes of hypocapnia
See Table 10.2.

Table 10.2 Common causes of hypocapnia

Hypoxaemia	A low arterial P_{O_2} especially when less than 8 kPa causes a compensatory increase in ventilatory drive, with resultant reduction in P_{CO_2}
Metabolic acidosis	Compensatory hyperventilation reduces arterial P_{CO_2}
CNS disorders	Subarachnoid haemorrhage, trauma, infection, tumours may cause hyperventilation by cerebral irritation
Drugs	Salicylates stimulate respiratory drive
Anxiety hyperventilation	Important to exclude the above before making this diagnosis

ASSESSMENT OF OXYGENATION

After examination of arterial P_{CO_2}, a patient's oxygenation should be assessed by examination of arterial P_{O_2} and haemoglobin saturation, S_aO_2.

ASSESSMENT OF ARTERIAL P_{O_2}

The oxygen cascade

> # Key definition
> - P_{O_2} Partial pressure of oxygen in atmospheric air, dry

Oxygen makes a journey from the atmosphere through the upper airway, alveoli, arterial blood, capillaries and tissues to the mitochondria. In a perfect system, P_{O_2} would be 21 kPa throughout the system, i.e. equal to its partial pressure in the atmosphere. With each transition along the pathway, however, there is a drop in P_{O_2}, which falls in a series of steps, called the oxygen cascade.

> **Physiology: P_{O_2} of atmospheric air, dry**
> The partial pressure of oxygen in the atmosphere at sea level is equal to the product of barometric pressure and the fractional

concentration of oxygen:

$$Po_2 = P_B \times F_IO_2$$
$$= 101.3 \times 0.21$$
$$= 21 \, kPa$$

where

P_B = atmospheric pressure = 101.3 kPa at sea level
F_IO_2 = fractional concentration of oxygen in air = 0.21.

Although the ultimate purpose of the respiratory system is to provide adequate oxygen to the tissues, they differ widely in their requirements and supply. As arterial blood is the same throughout the body and easy to sample, it provides a convenient means of assessing pulmonary function.

We will now consider the steps of the oxygen cascade from the atmosphere to blood.

Oxygen cascade 1: inspired gas
● P_IO_2 Partial pressure of oxygen in inspired gas, humidified

In the first step of the oxygen cascade, inspired air becomes humidified in the upper airway, so that it is fully saturated with water by the time it reaches the trachea.

Physiology: dilution of inspired O_2 by water vapour

When air enters the nose and oropharynx, it becomes saturated with water vapour. This dilutes all other alveolar gases by a factor of:

$$\text{Dilution factor} = \frac{\text{atmospheric pressure} - \text{partial pressure of water vapour}}{\text{atmospheric pressure}}$$

$$= \frac{101.3 - 6.3}{101.3} \quad \text{(partial pressure of water vapour} = 6.3 \, kPa)$$

$$= 0.95$$

The inspired P_IO_2 humidified is, therefore:

$$\mathbf{P_IO_2 = F_IO_2 \times P_B \times 0.95}$$
$$= 0.21 \times 101.3 \times 0.95$$
$$= 20\,kPa$$

where

P_IO_2 = *effective* inspired Po_2 (humidified)
F_IO_2 = fractional concentration of O_2 (dry)
P_B = barometric pressure = 101.3 kPa at sea level.

KEYPOINTS

- Atmospheric Po_2 (dry) is 21 kPa
- Inspired gas Po_2 (humidified) is 20 kPa

Oxygen cascade 2: alveolar gas

- P_AO_2 Partial pressure of oxygen in alveolar gas

On entering the alveoli, the inspired Po_2 drops further, to a level which may be calculated by the alveolar air equation.

Physiology: alveolar air equation

In the alveoli, O_2 is exchanged for CO_2. If CO_2 and O_2 are exchanged at a 1:1 ratio, the volume of O_2 consumed is replaced by an equal volume of CO_2 produced. Then

alveolar Po_2 + alveolar Pco_2 = inspired Po_2

As alveolar Pco_2 is approximately equal to arterial Pco_2:

alveolar Po_2 + arterial Pco_2 = inspired Po_2

Rearranging:

alveolar Po_2 = inspired Po_2 − arterial Pco_2
$$P_AO_2 = P_IO_2 - P_aCO_2$$

The ratio of CO_2 produced/O_2 consumed is governed by the respiratory quotient (R). Although equal to unity on a pure carbohydrate diet, 0.8 is a more typical value.

More accurately then:

$$P_AO_2 = P_IO_2 - P_aCO_2/0.8$$
$$P_AO_2 = P_IO_2 - 1.25\,P_aCO_2$$

This is a simplified form of the alveolar air equation.

Factors affecting alveolar Po_2

The alveolar air equation describes the factors which influence alveolar Po_2 and therefore arterial Po_2. These are:

- inspired Po_2
- ventilation: an increase in ventilation reduces alveolar Pco_2, thereby raising alveolar Po_2
- respiratory quotient (and, therefore, carbohydrate content of diet).

Alveolar Po_2 is closely related to arterial Po_2, the two values being within 2 kPa in healthy young subjects. Alveolar Po_2 is important because it may easily be calculated from the above equation and, from this, the difference between alveolar Po_2 and measured arterial Po_2 found. This gradient is a very useful index of how well the lungs are working, and gives more information than the arterial Po_2 alone (see 'Alveolar–arterial oxygen partial pressure difference').

Relationship between alveolar Po_2 and arterial Pco_2

From the alveolar air equation a simple graph may be drawn (Fig. 11.1; see p. 87). This graph is an approximation (in reality the line is curved) but a number of important points are illustrated as follows:

- For a given inspired concentration of oxygen (and R), there is only one possible arterial Pco_2 for each value of alveolar Po_2. The two alter as though on a pair of scales, with any reduction in one associated with an increase in the other.
- A patient with mild respiratory impairment may normalize Po_2 by increasing the minute volume of ventilation (by reducing alveolar Pco_2).

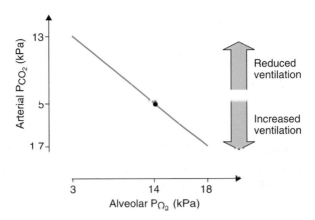

Fig. 11.1

Relationship between arterial P_{CO_2} and alveolar P_{O_2} breathing room air

This graph is an approximation, and in reality the line is curved. Certain principles are illustrated, however. The alveolar P_{O_2} and arterial P_{CO_2} are interdependent, as though on a pair of scales. An increase in one is associated with a reduction in the other. The point indicated corresponds to normal ventilation. From the graph it is seen that the highest alveolar P_{O_2} attainable breathing room air is limited by the extent to which arterial P_{CO_2} may fall. Likewise, the upper limit to which arterial P_{CO_2} can climb is constrained by the lowest P_{O_2} compatible with survival.

- Hypoventilation reduces oxygenation by causing an increase in alveolar P_{CO_2}. The accumulation of this gas then reduces the fractional concentration of oxygen present in the alveoli, and so its partial pressure, alveolar P_{O_2}. This is the mechanism of hypoxaemia in hypoventilation.
- The highest arterial P_{O_2} attainable breathing room air is determined by the limit to which alveolar (and so arterial) P_{CO_2} can fall. The lowest values of arterial P_{CO_2} recorded are around 1.7 kPa, which is reached in high-altitude mountaineers or extreme panic. In these high-ventilation states, alveolar P_{O_2} may reach 17–18 kPa. Because there is always a gradient between alveolar and arterial P_{O_2}, arterial P_{O_2} is limited to around 16 kPa.
- In respiratory failure, the maximum arterial P_{CO_2} that may be reached breathing room air is determined by the limit of

a patient's tolerance of hypoxaemia. If the arterial P_O_2 drops as low as 4 kPa, then alveolar (and so arterial) P_{CO_2} may climb as high as 12 kPa. Consciousness is lost in normal subjects, if arterial P_O_2 drops below about 3.5 kPa, but in chronically hypoxic patients or acclimatised mountaineers, this value may be as low as 2.5 kPa.

KEYPOINT

Hypoventilation causes both hypoxaemia and hypercapnia. When oxygen is used to correct hypoxaemia arising from hypoventilation, oxygenation may be maintained despite falling ventilation, allowing P_{CO_2} to climb catastrophically. P_{CO_2} must be monitored under these circumstances.

Clinical aspects: apnoeic respiration

If a subject becomes apnoeic after a period of breathing 100% oxygen, there is adequate oxygen in the lungs to maintain oxygenation for a considerable period. If airway patency is maintained and a continuous supply of oxygen provided, alveolar oxygenation may be maintained for up to one hour. As no ventilation occurs, however, alveolar P_{CO_2} rises by a rate of 0.4–0.8 kPa/min and its presence eventually 'dilutes' the oxygen until the alveolar P_O_2 falls. Deleterious hypercapnia would ensue, however, before this occurred.

Oxygen cascade 3: arterial blood

● P_aO_2 Partial pressure of oxygen in arterial blood
● $A–aP_O_2$ Alveolar–arterial P_O_2 difference

A further reduction in P_O_2 occurs between the alveoli and the arterial blood. This is an important concept, and the drop is called the alveolar–arterial oxygen partial pressure difference ($A–aP_O_2$). The normal arterial P_O_2 is between 10.6 kPa in the elderly and 13.3 kPa in the young.

This step of the oxygen cascade is where oxygenation becomes impaired in disease, and so is of great importance. A low arterial P_{O_2} is not, however, caused by failure of diffusion across the blood–gas barrier, but ventilation/perfusion mismatch, the subject of Chapter 12 'Distribution of ventilation and perfusion'.

Alveolar arterial oxygen partial pressure difference

We can gain information about the efficiency of gas exchange by considering the difference between the *measured arterial* P_{O_2} and the *calculated alveolar* P_{O_2} on which it depends. This difference is small in healthy subjects (up to 2 kPa in young adults breathing air).

Why calculate the A–aP_{O_2}?

Calculation of the alveolar–arterial gradient is a powerful tool, enabling evaluation of more complicated oxygenation problems. Because arterial P_{O_2} is a function of both ventilation and respiratory quotient (as well as $F_{I}O_2$), it has a range of normality. By calculating the alveolar–arterial gradient, we define more precise limits within which P_{O_2} should lie. This may be particularly helpful in the following:

- To unmask a subtle impairment of gas exchange, not otherwise clinically evident. This may be especially helpful in conditions with a normal chest X-ray, e.g. early interstitial lung disease or suspected pulmonary embolus.
- When a subject is hyperventilating or hypoventilating.
- When the $F_{I}O_2$ is other than 0.21.

KEYPOINT

The calculated alveolar P_{O_2} gives a predicted range for the arterial P_{O_2}, *which is specific to the subject's rate of ventilation.*

Calculation of alveolar–arterial partial pressure difference

The alveolar air equation as given above is accurate enough for bedside purposes and simple enough to be calculated mentally. The appropriate values of P_IO_2 and arterial PCO_2 are entered into the alveolar air equation. This gives a value for alveolar PO_2 from which the measured arterial PO_2 is subtracted. The difference between the two should be less than 2 kPa in young healthy subjects (see examples).

Example 1
A 25-year-old woman (non-smoker) comes to casualty complaining of shortness of breath that started suddenly. She appears anxious. The chest X-ray is normal. Arterial blood gas analysis shows that $PO_2 = 10.1$ kPa and $PCO_2 = 3.7$ kPa.

Question: Is this a panic attack?

$$P_IO_2 = 20 \text{ kPa (see 'Oxygen cascade 1')}$$

$$\text{Calculated alveolar } PO_2 = P_IO_2 - 1.25 \times PCO_2$$
$$= 20 - 4.5$$
$$= 15.5 \text{ kPa}$$

$$\text{Alveolar–arterial difference} = 15.5 - 10.1$$
$$= 5.4 \text{ kPa}$$

This woman is, therefore, significantly hypoxic for her rate of ventilation and pulmonary embolus should be suspected with the history given.

Example 2
You are asked to review a patient in casualty. He is known to have COPD having smoked 40/day for 40 years. He presents with shortness of breath increasing over the last few days. He was cyanosed on presentation, so a face-mask oxygen was applied (24%), and arterial blood gases measured:
$PO_2 = 17$ kPa and $PCO_2 = 8$ kPa.

$$\text{Effective inspired } P_IO_2 = 0.24 \times 101.3 \times 0.95$$
$$= 23 \text{ kPa}$$

$$\text{Calculated alveolar } PO_2 = P_IO_2 - 1.25 \times PCO_2$$
$$= 23 - 1.25 \times 8$$
$$= 13 \text{ kPa}$$

$$\text{Alveolar–arterial difference} = 13 - 17$$
$$= -4\,\text{kPa}$$

This is an impossibility. The F_I0_2 *must* have been greater than 24%.

Twenty-four per cent may have been the *estimated* dose of oxygen, administered using a flow-dependent oxygen mask instead of a Venturi mask. This method is notoriously unreliable and should not be accepted as an alternative to a Venturi mask in patients to whom F_I0_2 must be carefully regulated.

As a quick approximation, the sum of arterial Po_2 and Pco_2 cannot exceed the inspired oxygen concentration.

Example 3
A 50-year-old non-smoker is referred to the respiratory outpatient department with increasing shortness of breath, which is worse when lying. He is fully alert and conscious. Blood gases show: $Po_2 = 8\,\text{kPa}$ and $Pco_2 = 8\,\text{kPa}$.

$$\text{Calculated alveolar } Po_2 = P_I0_2 - 1.25 \times Pco_2$$
$$= 20 - 1.25 \times 8$$
$$= 10\,\text{kPa}$$

$$\text{Alveolar–arterial difference} = 10 - 8$$
$$= 2\,\text{kPa}$$

This man's gas exchange is normal. The problem here is hypoventilation, as indicated by the raised Pco_2. A neuromuscular problem causing diaphragmatic weakness should be suspected, especially given the history of orthopnoea. There is no evidence of respiratory impairment given by the blood gases.

What is a normal arterial Po_2?
Normal values of arterial Po_2
- The normal arterial Po_2 is difficult to define as it changes with age, posture, body mass index, and the concentration of oxygen in the inspired gas.

- While breathing air, a normal subject should have arterial P_{O_2} in the range 10.6 kPa in the elderly to 13.3 kPa in the young (see 'Closing capacity' in Chapter 6 for a discussion of the cause of this range).
- Any change in the ventilation results in a significant change in arterial P_{O_2} within 30 sec reflecting the small oxygen stores in the body. If breathing air, it takes only 10 sec to lose consciousness in the event of a circulatory arrest and life cannot be sustained for more than a few minutes.
- Hypoxaemia is when arterial P_{O_2} is less than 10 kPa.

Clinical aspects of oxygenation: chronic respiratory failure

In chronic respiratory failure, a convalescent arterial P_{O_2} of less than 7.3 kPa is an indication for long-term domiciliary oxygen therapy. This has been shown to prolong survival in respiratory failure. It may be considered with an arterial P_{O_2} in the range 7.3–8.0 kPa, if there is clinical evidence of pulmonary artery hypertension. Smokers should stop smoking prior to prescription, not least because of the fire hazard posed.

Is hypoxaemia caused by impairment of diffusion of oxygen?

Hypoxaemia is characterized by a measurable increase in the alveolar–arterial P_{O_2} difference. Although one intuitively expects this to be caused by impairment of diffusion across the blood–gas barrier, it is not so. A widened alveolar–arterial difference is invariably caused by poor matching of ventilation to perfusion.

Even in fibrotic lung disease, where the blood–gas barrier is abnormally thickened, the cause of resting hypoxaemia is abnormal shunting of blood through underventilated units, rather than diffusion impairment. Only on exercise does diffusion limitation become a significant factor in the pathogenesis of hypoxaemia. This is the subject of the next chapter 'Distribution of ventilation and perfusion'.

12

DISTRIBUTION OF VENTILATION AND PERFUSION

Physiology: normal $\dot{V}/\dot{Q}$ ratio

If ventilation and perfusion of all alveoli were uniform, taking the lungs as a whole, typical resting values would be 4 l/min for alveolar ventilation ($\dot{V}$) and 5 l/min for pulmonary blood flow ($\dot{Q}$). Thus the overall ventilation/perfusion ($\dot{V}/\dot{Q}$) ratio would be 4/5 = 0.8.

In young healthy adults, most alveoli have $\dot{V}/\dot{Q}$ ratios in the range of 0.5–2.0. In alveoli with $\dot{V}/\dot{Q}$ ratios in this range, efficient gas exchange takes place, so that pulmonary capillary blood leaving these alveoli has values of Po_2 and Pco_2 very close to those of the alveolar gas. Efficient gas-exchanging alveoli are described as 'ideal'.

$\dot{V}/\dot{Q}$ mismatch

In disease states, there are regional inhomogeneities in ventilation and perfusion. This causes the range of $\dot{V}/\dot{Q}$ ratios to be very much wider. Those alveoli with ratios outside the normal range are poor gas-exchangers.

Low $\dot{V}/\dot{Q}$

In the extreme case of alveoli with no ventilation but good perfusion, $\dot{V}/\dot{Q}$ is zero. Blood perfusing these alveoli is not exposed to alveolar gas, so its Pco_2 and Po_2 remains the same as mixed venous blood. This blood is effectively 'shunted', i.e. the effect is as though it has by-passed the lungs.

High $\dot{V}/\dot{Q}$

In the extreme case of alveoli with no perfusion but good ventilation, $\dot{V}/\dot{Q}$ has a value of infinity. Blood is not exposed to these alveoli, which represent dead space. Alveolar gas has the same composition as saturated air inspired.

KEYPOINTS

- Dead space: alveoli with poor perfusion are *dead space*. The effect of dead space is to reduce the alveolar ventilation, causing a tendency to hypercapnia.
- Alveoli with poor ventilation cause *shunt*. This is blood that effectively bypasses the lungs, causing hypoxaemia.

DEAD SPACE

Dead space is the volume of inspired gas in a breath which does not take part in gas exchange. This is more accurately called physiological dead space and is made up of:

- the anatomical dead space, which is the volume of the conducting airways and is approximately 150 ml in adults;
- the alveolar dead space, which is the volume of poorly-perfused alveoli (with high $\dot{V}/\dot{Q}$ or infinite $\dot{V}/\dot{Q}$). In healthy subjects, alveolar dead space is small.

Physiological dead space is the sum of alveolar and anatomical dead space. Physiological dead space varies with tidal volume but remains a relatively constant proportion. It is, therefore, often expressed as the ratio V_D/V_T and is normally approximately 0.3 (approximately 150 ml/500 ml).

The dead space may be measured using the Bohr equation.

Physiology: Bohr equation

Alveolar CO_2 from perfused units is diluted into the whole of the tidal volume during expiration. The volume of dead space can, therefore, be measured using a dilution method, with CO_2 as the tracer gas.

If no CO_2 is inspired:

quantity of CO_2 in alveoli = quantity of CO_2 in the tidal volume

Mean alveolar CO_2 concentration × alveolar volume
= Mixed expired CO_2 concentration × tidal volume

As partial pressure is proportional to fractional concentration:

$$P_ACO_2 \times V_A = P_{\bar{E}}CO_2 \times V_T$$

where

V_A = alveolar volume
V_T = tidal volume
$P_{\bar{E}}CO_2$ = partial pressure of CO_2 in mixed expiratory gas.

But
alveolar volume = tidal volume − anatomical dead space

$$V_A = V_T - V_D$$

Substituting:

$$P_ACO_2 (V_T - V_D) = P_{\bar{E}}CO_2 \times V_T$$

Rearranging:

$$\frac{V_D}{V_T} = \frac{P_ACO_2 - P_{\bar{E}}CO_2}{P_ACO_2}$$

This is the Bohr equation.

Solving the Bohr equation

Gas sampled at the end of expiration is representative of alveolar gas. The end-tidal P_{CO_2} may, therefore, be substituted for alveolar P_{CO_2}. This may be measured by infrared capnography. End-expiratory gas is itself a mixture of that from both perfused and non-perfused alveoli and is, therefore, representative of the total alveolar volume. Hence the V_D measured is the anatomical dead space.

> If the value for CO_2 concentration in the ideal alveoli were substituted in the above equation, it would represent only the volume of gas-exchanging units. As arterial P_{CO_2} is extremely close to the P_{CO_2} of ideal alveoli, if this value is substituted for alveolar P_{CO_2}, the physiological dead space is calculated.

For the causes of increased dead space, see Table 12.1.

Table 12.1 Causes of increased dead space

Cause	Comment
Age	Dead space increases with age
Emphysema	Destruction of alveolar septae results in space, which is ventilated but without pulmonary tissue, i.e. dead space. The effect is particularly pronounced if there are large bullae communicating with the bronchial tree
Pulmonary embolus	Occlusion of part of the pulmonary circulation increases the alveolar dead space
Acute lung injury and ARDS	May be associated with huge dead space, exceeding 70% of tidal volume
Anaesthesia	Dead space increases under anaesthesia
Low cardiac output	A shocked state results in pulmonary hypotension with inadequate alveolar perfusion and a large dead space

Effects of increased dead space

In practice, subjects with increased dead space maintain alveolar ventilation by increasing minute volume, thereby achieving a normal arterial P_{CO_2}. An increase in dead space is, therefore, an uncommon cause of ventilatory failure, unless it is huge or the patient tires.

Clinical aspects of dead space

A handy approximate measure of dead space is the arterial/end-tidal CO_2 difference. The latter is routinely measured by capnography when under anaesthesia. A difference of greater than $2 \, kPa$ indicates an abnormal alveolar dead space.

SHUNT AND VENOUS ADMIXTURE

Shunt refers to blood that either bypasses the lungs or passes through non-ventilated alveoli without becoming oxygenated.

In the normal subject, there is a small right to left shunt, equivalent to approximately 2% of cardiac output. This is caused by venous blood returning to the left heart through bronchial veins and the Thebesian veins.

Calculation of pulmonary shunt

In pulmonary disease, additional shunt is caused by blood that passes through under-ventilated alveoli, with low $\dot{V}/\dot{Q}$ ratios. Shunt is quantified, however, as the amount of blood that would have to perfuse *completely unventilated* alveoli (zero $\dot{V}/\dot{Q}$) to produce the observed arterial P_{O_2}. The resulting value, the proportion of cardiac output shunted in this way, is referred to as *venous admixture* (Fig. 12.1).

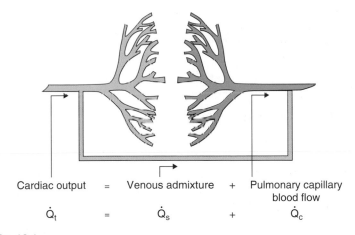

Cardiac output	=	Venous admixture	+	Pulmonary capillary blood flow
$\dot{Q}_t$	=	$\dot{Q}_s$	+	$\dot{Q}_c$

Fig. 12.1

Venous admixture

Most of the cardiac output passes through the pulmonary circulation ($\dot{Q}_c$). A proportion, which is small in health, bypasses the lungs. This is the venous admixture ($\dot{Q}_s$), which returns to the systemic circulation deoxygenated. The sum of the two flows is equal to the cardiac output ($\dot{Q}_t$).

t, total; s, shunt; c, capillary.

Venous admixture is calculated with the shunt equation.

Physiology: shunt equation (Fig. 12.1)

Considering blood flow through the heart:

The total cardiac output is comprised of oxygenated blood passing through alveoli with normal $\dot{V}/\dot{Q}$ ratios (pulmonary capillary blood flow) and deoxygenated blood, which is shunted (venous admixture). So we can write:

$$\text{cardiac output} = \text{pulmonary capillary blood flow} + \text{venous admixture}$$
$$\dot{Q}_t = \dot{Q}_c + \dot{Q}_s \tag{12.1}$$

Considering the flow of oxygen through the same channels:

The quantity of O_2 passing through the left ventricle:

$$C_aO_2 \times \dot{Q}_t = C'_cO_2 \times \dot{Q}_c + C_{\bar{v}}O_2 \times \dot{Q}_s \tag{12.2}$$

where:

C_aO_2 = arterial oxygen content
C'_cO_2 = pulmonary end-capillary oxygen content
$C_{\bar{v}}O_2$ = mixed venous oxygen content.

Rearranging (12.2) and substituting for $\dot{Q}_c$ from (12.1):

$$\frac{\dot{Q}_s}{\dot{Q}_t} = \frac{C'_cO_2 - C_aO_2}{C'_cO_2 - C_{\bar{v}}O_2}$$

This is the shunt equation.

Solving the shunt equation

- Arterial oxygen content can be determined from an arterial blood sample: $C_aO_2 = Hb \times S_aO_2 \times 1.31$ (see 'Oxygen content' in Chapter 13).
- Mixed venous oxygen content can be determined in a similar way from blood taken through a pulmonary artery catheter ($C_{\bar{v}}O_2 = Hb \times S_{\bar{v}}O_2 \times 1.31$). (*Venous blood is not entirely mixed until the pulmonary artery, as superior and inferior vena caval blood, and the coronary sinus blood all have different oxygen contents.*)

● Pulmonary end-capillary oxygen content cannot be measured directly, but can be derived from alveolar P_{O_2} calculated from the alveolar air equation and the dissociation curve.

For the causes of shunt, see Tables 12.2 and 12.3.

Table 12.2 Causes of pulmonary shunt

Cause	Comment
Pulmonary collapse	Collapsed lung is not ventilated but may still have significant blood flow, which returns to the heart deoxygenated
Pulmonary consolidation	Densely consolidated lung is very poorly ventilated
ALI and ARDS	ARDS is the most potent cause of hypoxaemia

Table 12.3 Causes of anatomical shunt

Cause	Comments
Bronchial and Thebesian veins	Deoxygenated blood from these vessels is returned to the left atrium
Congenital heart disease	Any right to left shunt, e.g. Eisenmenger syndrome secondary to atrial or ventricular septal defect, patent ductus arteriosus
Pulmonary arteriovenous malformation	May be a feature of hereditary haemorrhagic telangiectasia or may occur in isolation
Hepatopulmonary syndrome	This is hypoxaemia secondary to chronic liver disease. It is common (4–40% of chronic liver disease) and caused by intrapulmonary vascular dilatations, which allow blood to bypass the alveoli. The hypoxaemia is characteristically worse upright, improving when recumbent

Effects of venous admixture

The shunt equation tells us the proportion of cardiac output that must bypass the alveoli to cause a given degree of hypoxaemia. Although anatomical shunt, such as that caused by intracardiac shunt, originates in this way, pulmonary hypoxaemia is caused by blood returning to the heart from *under*ventilated alveolar units, rather than *non*-ventilated units. Pulmonary disease is characterized by a dispersion of the range of $\dot{V}/\dot{Q}$ ratios, so that an increased proportion have inadequate ventilation and return deoxygenated blood to the left atrium. Because end-capillary blood from normal alveolar units is already 100% saturated, an increase in ventilation or inspired oxygen concentration cannot compensate, and arterial hypoxaemia occurs. The effect of shunt on arterial P_{CO_2} in contrast is small.

Why is the response to oxygen variable in hypoxaemic patients?

In two extreme cases, pulmonary hypoxaemia could originate either from blood perfusing a large number of *marginally* underventilated units or a smaller number of completely *un*ventilated units. The importance of this distinction lies in the response a hypoxic subject is likely to make to supplementary oxygen.

When blood passes through completely unventilated units, there is minimal improvement in oxygenation when the F_IO_2 is increased. This is unusual in pulmonary hypoxaemia, and such a finding suggests the presence of an extrapulmonary or anatomical shunt.

KEYPOINTS

- An increase in dead space causes a tendency to hypercapnia. A subject can compensate for this to a large extent by hyperventilation.

- Shunt causes hypoxaemia but has little effect on P_{CO_2}. Only a limited correction to shunt can be made by hyperventilation.
- Anatomical shunt is absolute, i.e. $\dot{V}/\dot{Q}$ = zero. Therefore, increasing ventilation or F_IO_2 has little effect. Pulmonary shunt has an increased number of alveolar units with low $\dot{V}/\dot{Q}$ ratios but, as most receive some ventilation, an increase in ventilation or F_IO_2 improves oxygenation to some extent.
- Dense pulmonary consolidation or a collapsed lung are both potent causes of pulmonary shunt, where high inspired concentration of oxygen is likely to be necessary for adequate oxygenation.
- The normal value of shunt is around 2%. An increase to 10% would cause severe respiratory distress. Ventilatory assistance may be necessary when the shunt fraction is in the region of 15–25%.

Technique: measurement of clinical shunt

This is performed by asking a patient to breathe 100% oxygen. To achieve an F_IO_2 of 1.0, the patient breathes through a mouthpiece rather than a mask, so that no room air is entrained. Twenty minutes is usually sufficient time to ventilate alveolar units with low $\dot{V}/\dot{Q}$ ratios.

Arterial blood P_{O_2} is then measured, from which the shunt fraction can be calculated. In a normal subject, arterial P_{O_2} breathing 100% oxygen should be around 82 kPa. If the subject is asked to breathe with large tidal volumes, a value of around 84 kPa may be recorded. (see 'Closing volume' in Chapter 6). This corresponds to a shunt of approximately 2% of cardiac output.

The technique is not good for subjects with extensive air-trapping, in whom ventilation is so poorly distributed as to invalidate the technique.

Summary

Table 12.4.

Table 12.4 Causes of hypoxaemia by pathophysiology

Causes of hypoxaemia	Comments
Anatomical shunt	Caused by deoxygenated blood bypassing the lungs ($\dot{V}/\dot{Q} = 0$)
Pulmonary $\dot{V}/\dot{Q}$ mismatch	Caused by perfusion of poorly ventilated alveoli ($\dot{V}/\dot{Q} = 0 - 0.5$)
Hypoventilation	Raised alveolar P_{CO_2} reduces alveolar and arterial P_{O_2}
Alveolar–capillary diffusion impairment	This does *not* cause hypoxaemia in the resting subject, but contributes to exercise hypoxaemia in interstitial lung disease

13

ASSESSMENT OF HAEMOGLOBIN SATURATION

Key definitions
- S_aO_2 Percentage of arterial haemoglobin oxygenated, measured *in vitro*
- S_pO_2 Percentage of arterial haemoglobin oxygenated, measured with pulse oximetry

Physiology: oxyhaemoglobin dissociation curve

The carriage of O_2 is more complicated than that of CO_2. Whereas CO_2 is carried in physical solution in plasma, most oxygen is chemically bound to haemoglobin. The haemoglobin-bound oxygen is in equilibrium with a much smaller pool of oxygen in physical solution, the tension of which may be measured by blood gas analysis (arterial P_{O_2}).

The relationship between saturation of haemoglobin and the tension of oxygen in physical solution is non-linear and described by the familiar S-shaped haemoglobin-oxygen binding curve. Several important characteristics of oxygen transport are derived from the properties of the oxyhaemoglobin dissociation curve as listed below.

- Because the curve has a prolonged plateau, haemoglobin saturation is not significantly reduced by a drop in oxygen tension until arterial P_{O_2} falls below 10 kPa, so that blood oxygen content remains high under conditions of moderate hypoxaemia. Once on the steep part of the curve, any further drop in arterial P_{O_2} causes a significant reduction in arterial saturation (Fig. 13.1).

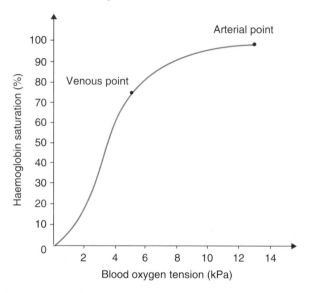

Fig. 13.1

Oxygen/haemoglobin dissociation curve

The curve indicates the percentage of haemoglobin saturated with oxygen for a given partial pressure of oxygen under normal conditions. The arterial point corresponds to oxygenation conditions found in normal arterial blood, the venous point to that of mixed venous blood. Owing to the sigmoidal shape of the curve, there may be a substantial fall in oxygen tension before saturation falls significantly.

● The curve shifts to the right in response to acidosis, raised arterial $P_{CO_2},$ raised temperature and raised intracellular levels of the intermediary metabolite 2,3-diphosphoglycerate (2,3-DGP). Likewise, a shift of the curve to the left occurs in response to alkalosis, or a reduction in arterial $P_{CO_2},$ temperature or 2,3-DPG (Fig. 13.2).

When haemoglobin is in the tissue capillary circulation, it is exposed to a greater concentration of the acidic gas CO_2 and

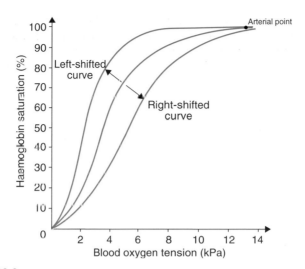

Fig. 13.2

Physiological shift of the oxyhaemoglobin dissociation curve

The oxyhaemoglobin dissociation curve is shifted to the right by an increase in hydrogen ion concentration, P_{CO_2}, 2,3-DPG and temperature. When the curve is right-shifted haemoglobin is less saturated at the same oxygen tension. As the curves are coincident at the arterial point, shift has very little effect on the affinity of arterial blood for oxygen. In the tissues, however, where blood is under venous conditions, the right-shift caused by increased carbon dioxide tension reduces affinity of haemoglobin for oxygen, facilitating release.

consequently the curve shifts to the right. Under these circumstances, haemoglobin has reduced affinity for oxygen (i.e. it carries less oxygen *at the same* P_{O_2}). This facilitates unloading of oxygen to the tissues. In the pulmonary circulation, where CO_2 concentration is lower, the curve shifts back to the left favouring oxygen binding and facilitating uptake.

This effect of pH on the affinity of oxygen is known as the Bohr effect.

What determines the amount of oxygen carried in blood?

The total amount of oxygen carried per volume of blood, or oxygen content, is determined as follows.

Physiology: oxygen content

Arterial oxygen content = haemoglobin concentration
$\times$ haemoglobin saturation
$\times$ oxygen-combining capacity
of haemoglobin

The oxygen-combining capacity of haemoglobin is experimentally determined to be 1.31 ml of oxygen per gram of haemoglobin.

Approximate normal values can, therefore, be calculated:

$$C_aO_2 = 15\,g/dl \times 0.97 \times 1.31\,ml/g = 19\,ml/dl$$

where C_aO_2 = arterial oxygen content.

To this a small extra contribution (of around 0.3 ml/dl) is made by oxygen in physical solution in plasma.

OXYGEN IN PHYSICAL SOLUTION

- At normal arterial P_{O_2}, the oxygen in physical solution is about 0.3 ml/dl. Under these circumstances, it makes a negligible contribution to oxygen delivery. When breathing 100% oxygen this may rise to 2 ml/dl.
- In a hyperbaric chamber, a patient may breathe 100% oxygen at 3 atmospheres. Under these conditions, the concentration of oxygen in physical solution rises to 6 ml/dl. This alone is sufficient to meet the metabolic needs of the tissues, so that venous blood returns to the heart fully saturated. This hyperoxic environment is toxic to anaerobic bacteria and is used to treat necrotizing soft tissue infections.

How does the arterial P_{O_2} affect the quantity of oxygen carried in blood?

Arterial P_{O_2} only affects blood oxygen content indirectly by its effect on haemoglobin–oxygen binding.

What is the effect of anaemia?

In anaemia, haemoglobin concentration and consequently oxygen content are reduced. There is no effect on the oxygen saturation of the haemoglobin present (S_aO_2), or on the arterial Po_2.

Oxygen delivery

> **Physiology: oxygen delivery**
>
> This is the quantity of oxygen made available to the body in one minute.
>
> $$O_2 \text{ delivery} = \text{cardiac output} \times \text{arterial oxygen content}$$
>
> Therefore
>
> $$O_2 \text{ delivery} = \text{cardiac output} \times \text{haemoglobin concentration} \\ \times \text{haemoglobin saturation} \\ \times \text{oxygen-carrying capacity of haemoglobin}$$
>
> $$\dot{D}o_2 = \dot{Q} \times Hb \times S_aO_2 \times 1.31$$
>
> where $\dot{D}o_2$ = oxygen delivery.

> ## KEYPOINTS
>
> ● Oxygen delivery is proportional to three variables: cardiac output, haemoglobin concentration and haemoglobin saturation.
> ● It is haemoglobin saturation (rather than arterial Po_2) that determines oxygen content and, therefore, oxygen delivery.

Normal values
● Arterial oxygen content, C_aO_2
   Around 19 ml of oxygen are carried in each 100 ml of blood
● Arterial oxygen saturation, S_aO_2
   Normal lungs should provide enough oxygen to saturate all haemoglobin passing through the pulmonary circulation. Mixing of this with venous blood from the bronchial

circulation and Thebesian veins reduces normal arterial saturation to 97%.

● Oxygen delivery, $\dot{D}o_2$
Around 1000 ml of oxygen are delivered to tissues every minute under resting conditions.

● Oxygen consumption, $\dot{V}o_2$
In adults at rest, about 250 ml/min of oxygen are used giving an extraction of 25%. The remaining oxygen serves as an important reserve, which may be utilized under conditions of exercise or stress, when extraction may rise to around 75%.

● Mixed venous saturation, $S_{\bar{v}}o_2$
Resting mixed venous saturation is in the region of 70–75%. Different tissues extract differing proportions of the arterial oxygen content, so that venous saturation varies around the body.

Pulse oximetry (S_po_2)

Reduced haemoglobin is bluish in colour, giving the hypoxic patient a cyanotic appearance. To be clinically detectable, there must be 5 g/dl of reduced haemoglobin, equating to an S_ao_2 of 67% (if Hb is 15 g/dl). This makes cyanosis a late and unreliable sign of hypoxaemia.

Pulse oximetry quantifies arterial blood colour by its light absorption, measured during arterial pulsation. From this, the proportion of haemoglobin combined with oxygen (the oxygen saturation) is derived. The measurement is made non-invasively using a probe attached to the finger, ear or nasal septum. It may be performed at the bedside, during exercise testing, in the clinic or during a home sleep study. In addition to pulse rate and continuous oxygen saturation, better oximeters provide a peripheral pulse waveform.

PITFALL

A significant reduction in arterial Po_2 produces only a minimal reduction in oxygen saturation until the steeper portion of the oxygen dissociation curve is encountered, i.e. a Po_2 of below 10 kPa or saturation of 94%. Haemoglobin saturation is, therefore, a less sensitive measure of oxygenation than arterial Po_2 and reliance upon it may miss clinically significant hypoxaemia.

Measurement of S_pO_2

Inaccurate pulse oximeter readings may arise in the following circumstances.

● Variant haemoglobins, or a combination of haemoglobin with other moieties:
  ● Inaccurate readings are obtained with Hb types other than HbA, HbF and HbS.
  ● Presence of carboxyhaemoglobin and methaemoglobin
● Poor pulse signal; this may be indicated by a pulse waveform which is damped or even lost.
  ● Poor peripheral perfusion caused by hypotension or cold hands.
  ● Dark nail varnish, false nails.
  ● Poor contact of the probe.
  ● Patient movement.

The reading is not affected by skin pigmentation.

PITFALL

A low saturation reading should prompt a check of the pulse signal. If a good waveform is displayed, transduction problems are unlikely and one should assume the patient is really hypoxaemic, until proven otherwise. Oximeters that display a waveform are preferred for this reason.

A low S_pO_2 reading together with a clean pulse waveform indicates that the patient is really hypoxaemic.

> ## KEYPOINTS
>
> ● Pulse oximetry is non-invasive and remarkably safe. It is an essential first-line assessment of the breathless patient.
> ● Saturation gives no information about P_{CO_2} or ventilation.

Clinical aspects of pulse oximetry: carbon monoxide poisoning

Carbon monoxide poisoning must be quickly recognized, but is frequently unsuspected. Carbon monoxide causes a low arterial oxygen saturation in the presence of a well-maintained arterial P_{O_2}. This occurs despite exposure of pulmonary capillary blood to normal alveolar pressures of O_2 because carbon monoxide has far greater affinity for haemoglobin and displaces oxygen from binding sites. Haemoglobin saturation is, therefore, reduced despite preservation of arterial P_{O_2}.

The carbon monoxide molecule also has a direct neurotoxic effect on the CNS, a cardinal sign of which is ataxia. Other symptoms are non-specific and include nausea, vomiting, headache, fits and drowsiness, which progresses to coma.

Immediate management should be with 100% oxygen. Carboxyhaemoglobin concentration may be measured on blood gas analysers, and any case with more than 20% carboxyhaemoglobinaemia and/or neurological symptoms should be discussed with the regional hyperbaric unit.

> ## PITFALL
>
> Pulse oximetry may give a misleadingly high reading of haemoglobin oxygenation in carbon monoxide poisoning, as it cannot distinguish between oxyhaemoglobin and carboxyhaemoglobin. A direct measurement of S_aO_2 from a blood gas analyser is needed.

14

RESPIRATION AND ACID-BASE BALANCE

Metabolism is an oxidative process, the products of which subject any organism to acidosis. Maintenance of acid/base balance is essential for life as many biochemical processes are pH-dependent.

Physiology: carriage of CO_2

CO_2 is a ubiquitous product of oxidative metabolism and combines with water to form carbonic acid (14.1):

$$CO_2 + H_2O \xrightarrow{\text{CA}} H_2CO_3 \rightleftharpoons H^+ + HCO_3^-$$

$$(14.1) \qquad\qquad (14.2)$$

The hydration (14.1) is sluggish unless catalysed by carbonic anhydrase (CA). CO_2 formed in the tissues enters the blood and diffuses into erythrocytes, where carbonic anhydrase is present in abundance. Nonetheless, the equilibrium lies far to the left.

Carbonic acid formed from this hydration dissociates (14.2) into its conjugate base (bicarbonate) and the hydrogen ion. The extent of the dissociation and, therefore, strength of the acid is expressed as the K_a. A weak acid such as carbonic is largely undissociated, so that

---

the equilibrium of (14.2) is also to the left.

$$K_a = \frac{[H^+][HCO_3^-]}{[H_2CO_3]}$$

Rearranging:

$$[H^+] = \frac{K_a[H_2CO_3]}{[HCO_3^-]}$$

Taking logs and switching signs:

$$pH = pK_a + \log\frac{[HCO_3^-]}{[H_2CO_3]}$$

The concentration of H_2CO_3 is difficult to measure, may be calculated from concentration of CO_2 in solution and its $K_{hydration}$. Arterial P_{CO_2} can, therefore, be substituted for $[CO_2]$ with the appropriate conversion factor. We then say:

$$pH = 6.1 + \log\frac{[HCO_3^-]}{\alpha P_a CO_2}$$

where [ ] denotes concentration in solution and α is a constant. This is the Henderson–Hasselbalch equation.

KEYPOINTS

- We see from the equation that for any pH value, there is always the same ratio of HCO_3^- to CO_2 species. At physiological pH, this is always 20:1, regardless of the concentrations of either.
- If either P_{CO_2} or HCO_3^- becomes deranged, physiological compensation occurs by adjustment of the other parameter, so preserving the ratio and maintaining pH.

CLASSIFICATION OF ACID–BASE DISORDERS

Key definitions
- pH   The negative log of the hydrogen ion concentration (normal range 7.38–7.42).
- $[H^+]$ Hydrogen ion concentration (normal range 38–42 nmol/l).

Metabolic disorder

Metabolic acidosis is caused by addition of an acid other than CO_2 to body fluid, (usually lactic acid, ketones or uraemic metabolites) or by excessive loss of bicarbonate. In either situation $[HCO_3^-]$ is reduced. The lungs compensate by increasing ventilation and eliminating CO_2 in an attempt to restore the HCO_3^-/CO_2 ratio. See Tables 14.1 and 14.2 for common causes of metabolic acidosis and alkalosis.

Metabolic alkalosis is caused pathologically by loss of H^+ from the system. Alkalosis may occur iatrogenically if excessive HCO_3^- is administered. The result of either is an increase in plasma HCO_3^-. Compensation occurs by a reduction

Table 14.1 Common causes of metabolic acidosis

Diabetic ketoacidosis
Renal failure
Bicarbonate-losing diarrhoea
Salicylate poisoning
Type A lactic acidosis (tissue hypoperfusion, e.g. shock, cardiac arrest)
Type B lactic acidosis (no tissue hypoperfusion, e.g. liver failure, diabetes mellitus)

Table 14.2 Common causes of metabolic alkalosis

Loss of gastric acid, i.e. vomiting or nasogastric drainage
Excessive bicarbonate administration

in ventilation, increasing P_{CO_2} and again restoring the HCO_3^-/CO_2 ratio and pH.

There is limited scope for respiratory compensation of metabolic alkalosis without compromising oxygenation by hypoventilation, so that the arterial P_{CO_2} seldom rises above 7.5 kPa, unless supplementary oxygen is given.

KEYPOINTS

- *Compensation* does not restore *normality*, but matches abnormal HCO_3^- concentration with an abnormal P_{CO_2}. Normality may only be restored by metabolic correction.
- Respiratory compensation is invariably partial rather than total, i.e. pH returns *toward* the physiologically normal state, but will not quite reach it.

Respiratory disorder

In respiratory alkalosis or acidosis, P_{CO_2} is deranged by hyperventilation or hypoventilation, respectively. The kidney compensates by adjusting bicarbonate to restore the HCO_3^-/P_{CO_2} ratio. Metabolic compensation takes days rather than the hours taken for respiratory compensation. In a compensatory response to respiratory alkalosis, the bicarbonate seldom falls below 18 mmol/l acutely or 15 mmol/l chronically.

PITFALL

Attempting to correct respiratory alkalosis without first ruling out hypoxaemia, pulmonary embolism and sepsis. Treatment of respiratory alkalosis is correction of the primary problem.

The causes of respiratory acidosis are those of hypercapnia (Table 10.1) and the causes of respiratory alkalosis are those of hypocapnia (Table 10.2). See 'Clinical aspects of arterial P_{CO_2}' in Chapter 10.

Mixed disorders

Both respiratory and metabolic disorders may coexist. Careful examination is needed not to overlook an additional component of the disorder. This may be identified if both bicarbonate and P_{CO_2} are changed in the direction of the pH abnormality, rather than one compensating the other.

DERIVED PARAMETERS

Bicarbonate and base excess are calculated from pH and P_{CO_2}. They yield no extra information, but offer another way of looking at the same data.

Standard bicarbonate

The standard bicarbonate is the value of arterial bicarbonate that would be measured with the P_{CO_2} clamped at 5.3 kPa. This standardizes the measuring conditions to eliminate any respiratory contribution to the bicarbonate level.

The normal standard bicarbonate is 24 mmol/l. The arterial bicarbonate is low in metabolic acidosis and raised in metabolic alkalosis.

Base excess

The base excess is the quantity of base or acid needed to titrate one litre of blood to pH 7.4, with the P_{CO_2} held constant at 5.3 kPa (40 mmHg). By clamping the P_{CO_2} at a normal value, it is a means of quantifying the metabolic derangement. The normal value is from −2.5 to 2.5 mmol/l.

In the context of an acidosis, a negative base excess (base deficit) indicates there is a metabolic component. Likewise, a positive base excess indicates a metabolic component to an alkalosis.

EVALUATION OF ACID/BASE DISORDER

1 First look at the pH or $[H^+]$. Is there acidosis or alkalosis?
   - Acidosis   pH < 7.35
   - Alkalosis   pH > 7.45
2 Then look at the arterial P_{CO_2}, as this indicates the origin of
   the disorder. The arterial P_{CO_2} is raised in respiratory
   acidosis and low in respiratory alkalosis.
   - Respiratory acidosis   arterial $P_{CO_2} > 6.0$ kPa
   - Respiratory alkalosis   arterial $P_{CO_2} < 4.7$ kPa
   If the change in arterial P_{CO_2} is in the direction of the pH
   abnormality, there is a respiratory component of the
   disorder. If not, the change in P_{CO_2} is compensatory, and the
   primary disorder is metabolic.
3 Look at the bicarbonate. Does the bicarbonate change in a
   direction that explains the pH change? If so, there is a
   metabolic component to the disorder. If not, the change is
   compensatory.
   - Metabolic acidosis   arterial bicarbonate < 22 mmol/l
   - Metabolic alkalosis   arterial bicarbonate > 26 mmol/l
4 A normal pH does not exclude an acid–base disorder, as
   compensation may have completely corrected an underlying
   acidotic or alkalotic tendency. If the pH is normal, check the
   P_{CO_2}. If this is abnormal, there is a compensated state. This
   then poses a difficult question: is this a case of complete
   respiratory compensation for a metabolic disorder or
   vice versa? As respiratory compensation is rarely complete,
   it is more likely to represent complete metabolic
   compensation of a respiratory disorder.

KEYPOINTS

- The primary abnormality is that which explains the observed
  pH change.
- Respiratory compensation is invariably incomplete.

Example 1

A man comes to casualty complaining of increased shortness of breath. He stopped smoking 10 per day 20 years ago.

Arterial blood gases:

- pH 7.33
- P_{O_2} 8 kPa
- P_{CO_2} 7.3 kPa
- Bicarbonate 26 mmol/l
- Base excess +3 mmol/l.

Comment on the acid–base status.

- There is acidosis.
- The P_{CO_2} is raised, indicating that it is respiratory in origin.
- The bicarbonate is high/normal, i.e. in the opposite sense to the pH change. There is, therefore, no coexisting metabolic component.
- As the rise in CO_2 has caused marked acidosis, we can see that little metabolic compensation has taken place and the rise in P_{CO_2} is of acute onset.

Example 2

A woman comes into casualty with two days increasing shortness of breath and cough productive of green sputum. She smokes 30 per day.

Arterial blood gases (measured breathing air):

- pH 7.38
- P_{O_2} 6 kPa
- P_{CO_2} 7 kPa
- Bicarbonate 30 mmol/l
- Base excess +7 mmol/l.

Comment on the acid–base status.

- The pH is normal.
- There is marked hypoxaemia and respiratory failure.

- The P_{CO_2} is raised. As the pH is normal, the state is compensated and of long-standing, i.e. the patient has chronic respiratory failure.
- The high bicarbonate confirms metabolic compensation.

Example 3

A boy presents to casualty in a rather drowsy state. He is breathing deeply.

Arterial blood gases (on air):

- pH 7.28
- P_{O_2} 14 kPa
- P_{CO_2} 3.8 kPa
- Bicarbonate 17 mmol/l
- Base excess -12 mmol/l.

Comment on the acid–base status.

- There is an acidosis.
- The P_{CO_2} is low, indicating that this is a metabolic disorder.
- The low bicarbonate confirms a metabolic origin. This is metabolic acidosis, with a degree of respiratory compensation.

Example 4

A patient has a respiratory arrest on the ward, from which he is quickly resuscitated. The following blood gases are made, while the patient is breathing high-concentration oxygen.

Arterial blood gases:

- pH 7.20
- P_{O_2} 20 kPa
- P_{CO_2} 8 kPa
- Base excess -9 mmol/l
- Bicarbonate 15 mmol/l

Comment on the acid–base status.

- There is severe acidosis.

- The P_{CO_2} is raised indicating a respiratory contribution.
- The bicarbonate is low, indicating an additional metabolic contribution.
- This is a mixed respiratory and metabolic acidosis. Metabolic acidosis is common after a period of circulatory arrest.

Clinical aspects of acid–base disorders

- Acidosis in critically ill patients is often caused by lactate production, secondary to failure of tissue perfusion and/or oxygen uptake. The onset of lactic acidosis in a sick patient is a grave sign, which is frequently overlooked. Identification of a metabolic acidosis on blood gas measurements should prompt a lactate measurement (many blood gas analysers perform this). Significant metabolic acidosis should prompt a discussion with the intensive care unit. The base deficit is a useful way of quantifying a metabolic acidosis.
- The bicarbonate is useful for gaining information about the chronicity of a raised P_{CO_2}. A chronic CO_2 retainer has a raised bicarbonate, as the kidney retains this ion to buffer the respiratory acidosis.
- A raised venous bicarbonate is a common incidental finding on routine electrolyte measurement. Compensation for chronic CO_2 retention is one of the commonest causes. (Diuretic use is another.)

PART

III

EXERCISE TESTING

15

DISABILITY ASSESSMENT TESTS

These are performed in patients with a known diagnosis, to assess the level of disability. Pulse oximetry may be used in either. The tests may be useful to provide objective assessment of response to treatment or rehabilitation.

SIX-MINUTE WALK

The subject is asked to walk for six minutes and to go as far as possible in that time. The result is expressed as the distance covered and the time taken. No encouragement should be given, as this may alter the results obtained.

SHUTTLE WALK TEST

In this test the subject is asked to walk between two cones placed ten metres apart. The subject is asked to reach the cone by the time a bleep is sounded. The bleeps occur at progressively shorter intervals.

Both tests are well validated and widely used. Reproducibility of the shuttle test is better, whereas the six-minute walk may better reflect the activities of daily living.

16

LIMITED EXERCISE TESTING WITH SATURATION MONITORING

This may be performed informally on the ward or in outpatients by attaching a probe to a patient's finger, and walking with them up a flight of stairs or along a corridor. Alternatively, the exercise may be performed according to a protocol, such as the six-minute walk or shuttle test.

● Significant desaturation during exercise is always abnormal.
● Desaturation on exercise is often the first sign of disease.

Exercise testing is a useful test for detection of lung disease before it is radiologically evident, e.g. early fibrosis, *Pneumocystis carinii* pneumonia or pulmonary vascular disease. Patients with airway disease and those with interstitial disease may desaturate on exercise. In interstitial disease, however, desaturation is incremental throughout exercise, worsening as exercise progresses. This is because, *under exercising conditions*, the alveolar-capillary thickening found in interstitial lung disease impairs diffusion to such a degree that it reduces oxygenation.

Definitive measurements of saturation require blood gas analysis of arterial specimens taken at baseline and peak exercise, as movement artefact degrades the signal from a pulse oximetry probe. Pulse oximetry during exercise may be extremely useful, however, as a screening procedure.

KEYPOINT

Impairment of resting oxygenation is a relatively insensitive sign of disease. Performing a limited exercise test may unmask a latent impairment.

17

MAXIMAL CARDIORESPIRATORY TESTING

This is an extensive area and the subject of many textbooks in its own right. Only an outline is presented.

Key definitions

- $\dot{V}_{O_2}$ Rate of oxygen consumption.
  An index of the work being done.

- $\dot{V}_{O_2max}$ Rate of oxygen consumption at maximum exercise attainable.
  This is a measure of a subject's maximum physical performance and overall fitness.

- V_{CO_2} Rate of carbon dioxide production.

- MVV   Measured maximum voluntary ventilation
  The volume exhaled during a short period of rapid forced breathing.

- $\dot{V}_{Emax}$ Ventilation at maximal exercise.

- $\dot{V}_{O_{Emax\ pred}}$ The predicted maximum ventilatory capacity on exercise, extrapolated from MVV or FEV_1.

LIMITATIONS TO EXERCISE PERFORMANCE

In maximal testing, the aim is to exercise a subject to close to the limit of their capacity, to obtain maximum performance indicators of cardiorespiratory function. The normal subject is limited by the capacity of the skeletal musculature to utilize oxygen rather than cardiac or pulmonary oxygen delivery factors.

> ## KEYPOINT
>
> Early attainment of maximal values of either cardiac or respiratory parameters indicates that disease in that system is the overall limitation to exercise performance.

Physiology: normal response to exercise

Cardiac output rises from its resting rate of 5 l/min to a maximum of around 20 l/min. At light workloads, there is increased stroke volume (from a normal baseline of around 80 ml up to around 110 ml) and heart rate. Thereafter, further demand is met by increasing heart rate alone.

Systolic blood pressure rises from 120 mmHg to around 200–250 mmHg. Diastolic blood pressure rises by 10–15 mmHg or less.

Ventilation also increases from its resting rate of 5–10 l/min to around 200 l/min in a conditioned subject. At low and moderate workloads, the increase is accommodated by raising tidal volume until V_T is approximately 65% of VC. After this, further demand is met by increasing respiratory rate up to a maximum of around 60/min (Fig. 17.1; see p. 131).

The increase in ventilation is not enough to meet the needs of maximum exercise. Further capacity is provided by extracting a greater proportion of the oxygen content of blood than under resting conditions and beyond this by anaerobic metabolism.

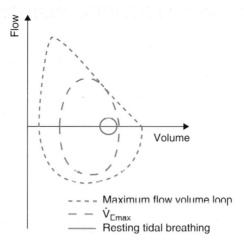

----- Maximum flow volume loop
-- -- $\dot{V}_{Emax}$
——— Resting tidal breathing

Fig. 17.1

Tidal loop and $\dot{V}_{Fmax}$

The inner circular loop is the flow volume trace of a resting subject taking normal tidal breaths, i.e. normal breathing. The outer dotted loop is a forced expiratory and inspiratory manoeuvre, i.e. normal maximal flow volume loop. This is an artificial manoeuvre and is never physiologically performed, even in the most severe exertion. The middle dashed loop is of a person at peak exercise. The tidal volumes used by a subject at peak exercise are about half vital capacity. Flow velocity is at its physiological maximum at only one point, where the $\dot{V}_{Emax}$ curve touches the MEFV curve.

In pulmonary exercise testing, expired gas is collected via a face mask, and its volume and CO_2 and O_2 concentration are measured. Oxygen consumption ($\dot{V}O_2$) is a direct index of the work being done. The work level attained at maximum exercise is indicated by $\dot{V}O_{2max}$. $\dot{V}O_2$ increases from approximately 250 ml/min at rest to 4 l/min in trained subjects at peak exercise.

Why perform cardiopulmonary exercise testing?

1   Exercising a subject to their maximum capacity allows a
    detailed assessment of their physiological state. This may be

useful to establish normality or otherwise, when the patient has a conviction that they are breathless and all other tests have proved normal.

2 Exercise testing may be useful where there is established reduction to exercise tolerance, and is not clear whether this is due to cardiac, pulmonary or other disease.

3 As part of a detailed assessment prior to transplantation or other major surgery.

4 To establish the relative contribution of different problems in a patient with cardiac and pulmonary disease.

Exercise impairment is measured by comparison of a subject's measured $\dot{V}_{O_{2max}}$ to the value predicted for their age, weight and gender. A value of less than 80% of predicted represents a significant impairment.

Ventilatory reserve

Maximum voluntary ventilation is a test of lung function in which the subject is asked to breathe in and out as rapidly and deeply as possible for 15 sec. From this, the theoretical maximum ventilatory capacity on exercise ($\dot{V}_{Emax\ pred}$) may be extrapolated[1].

The measured maximum ventilatory capacity ($\dot{V}_{Emax}$) is a subject's minute ventilation when at the limit of their exercise tolerance. It is the power of skeletal muscle, however, rather than ventilation that is the limiting factor to exercise in a normal subject. At peak exercise, $\dot{V}_{Emax}$ is always less than 70% of $\dot{V}_{Emax\ pred}$ in normal subjects.

The ventilatory reserve is $\dot{V}_{Emax\ pred} - \dot{V}_{Emax}$.

- A ventilatory reserve of less than 11 l/min suggests that respiratory function is limiting exercise capacity.

---

[1] MVV was formerly used as a laboratory test of lung function but is now used less often, as it is principally affected by airflow limitation, which is more easily assessed by simple spirometry. It is physically very demanding and unpleasant to perform because of the alkalosis induced. ($\dot{V}_{Emax\ pred}$ may also be predicted from FEV_1.)

- In subjects with ventilatory limitation to exercise, minute ventilation may reach 80% of $\dot{V}_{Emax\ pred}$ at peak exercise.
- The sensation of breathlessness occurs when $\dot{V}_E$ approaches 25% of $\dot{V}_{Emax\ pred}$. Only conditioned athletes can *sustain* a ventilation greater than 60% $\dot{V}_{Emax\ pred}$.

Heart rate reserve

An individual's maximum predicted heart rate is given by the equation:

$$HR_{max\ pred} = 220 - age$$

Greater than 85% $HR_{max\ pred}$ should be attained in any maximal exercise study. Failure to do so may occur in subjects with ventilatory limitation to exercise or those making poor effort. The heart rate reserve is the difference between the maximum predicted heart rate and that attained at peak exercise:

$$Heart\ rate\ reserve = HR_{max\ pred} - HR_{max\ ex}$$

A heart rate reserve of less than 15 beats/min suggests that cardiac function is limiting exercise capacity.

Lactate threshold

During incremental exercise, a sharp increase in arterial blood lactate occurs at a point known as the lactate threshold (Fig. 17.2; see p. 134). At this point anaerobic metabolism begins to supplement aerobic metabolism in providing energy for exercise. This point is also marked by an increase in the respiratory quotient, as CO_2 is produced without oxygen consumption. As anaerobic metabolism increases, the respiratory quotient rises to greater than unity.

The anaerobic threshold is raised by training, as skeletal muscles become more efficient at uptake and utilization of oxygen.

- Failure to reach the lactate threshold may occur in respiratory disease or a poorly-motivated subject. Lactate threshold is normally reached at 40–60% of $\dot{V}o_{2max}$.

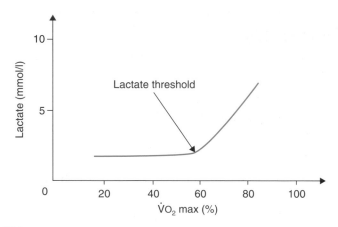

Fig. 17.2

Lactate threshold

As exercise increases, a point is reached at which aerobic metabolism can no longer keep pace with the energy demand. The circulating lactate level starts to rise steeply, as anaerobic metabolism supervenes. The inflection point in the curve is the lactate threshold. The trained subject reaches this point at a greater intensity of exercise and tolerates lactic acidaemia better than the unfit. A lactate level above about 10 mmol/l is intolerable to all but the trained athlete.

● A lactate threshold of less than 40% $\dot{V}o_{2max}$ is seen in cardiac disease but may also occur in the very unfit subject.
● Lactic acidosis becomes intolerable to an exercising subject and limits the endurance of maximal exercise when arterial concentration reaches around 10 mmol/l. Trained athletes can tolerate higher concentrations of lactate of around 20 mmol/l.
● A failure to produce lactate is the hallmark of McArdles disease.

Summary

Indicators that ventilation is the limiting factor in peak exercise:

- $\dot{V}_{Emax} > 80\%$ $\dot{V}_{Emax\ pred}$
- Ventilatory reserve < 11 l/min
- Desaturation
- Lactate threshold not reached.

Indicators that cardiac performance is the limiting factor in peak exercise:

- Heart rate reserve < 15 beats/min
- Lactate threshold occurring at less than 40% of predicted $\dot{V}_{O_{2max}}$.

PART

CHARACTERISTIC PATTERNS OF ABNORMALITY BY DISEASE

The most appropriate tests for a condition are indicated in bold.

ASTHMA

FEV_1/FVC	Reduced	(Episodic, and may be normal when convalescent, diurnal variation typical)
Peak flow	Reduced	Ditto
RV/TLC	Increased	
K_{CO}	Normal	May be helpful to distinguish from COPD
Flow volume loop	**Concavity of descending curve**	

COPD

FEV_1/FVC	Less than 0.7
Peak flow	Reduced

Reversibility	May be present, but normal spirometric values not attainable
TLC	Usually preserved; may be increased
RV/TLV	Always increased
TL_{CO}	Reduced
K_{CO}	Reduced
Flow volume loop	Early: concavity of descending curve Later: reduction of PEF
ABG	Type one or two respiratory failure when severe (FEV_1 usually less than 1 l at this stage)

LARGE AIRWAY OBSTRUCTION

FEV_1/FVC	Often preserved; may be reduced
Peak flow	Reduced, more so than FEV_1
Flow volume loop	Characteristic: extrathoracic obstruction-flattening of inspiratory curve, intrathoracic obstruction-flattening of expiratory curve

INTERSTITIAL LUNG DISEASE

FEV_1/FVC	Normal; may be increased
FVC	Reduced
Peak flow	Normal at first, then reduced
TLC	Reduced
TL_{CO}	Reduced
K_{CO}	Reduced (may be preserved in sarcoid or early CFA)
Flow volume loop	Early: increased slope of descending curve Reduced vital capacity and peak flow
ABG	Arterial Po_2 may be normal initially Alveolar-arterial Po_2 difference gradient increased Desaturation on exertion may be more sensitive than resting gases

SARCOIDOSIS

As other interstitial lung disease, but

FEV_1/FVC	May be reduced (a minority of patients have coexisting airflow limitation, possibly due to granulomatous infiltration of airways)
TL_{CO}	Reduced
K_{CO}	Tends to be relatively preserved

MUSCLE WEAKNESS

FEV_1/FVC	Often preserved; may be reduced
FVC	Reduced, especially supine
Peak flow	Reduced
RV	Increased or normal
TL_{CO}	Slightly reduced
K_{CO}	Greatly increased (differentiates from small, poorly compliant lungs, where K_{CO} is reduced)
Flow volume loop	Peak flow delayed and reduced, reduced MIFV curve
ABG	Type 2 respiratory failure occurs late; CO_2 may be raised in the morning before being raised throughout the day Alveolar-arterial Po_2 difference gradient usually normal

CHEST WALL STIFFNESS (e.g. PLEURAL DISEASE)

FEV_1/FVC	Preserved
TLC	Reduced

ANAEMIA

FEV_1/FVC	Normal
Peak flow	Normal

TLC	Normal
RV	Normal
TL_{CO}	Normal when corrected
K_{CO}	Normal when corrected
ABG	Normal
Saturation	Normal
Haemoglobin	Reduced

CARBON MONOXIDE POISONING

Pulse oximetry S_pO_2	Spuriously normal
Directly measured S_aO_2	Reduced
Arterial PO_2	Normal
Carboxyhaemoglobin	Raised

RECURRENT PULMONARY EMBOLI

FEV_1/FVC	Normal
TLC	Normal
RV	Normal
TL_{CO}	May be low or normal
K_{CO}	May be low or normal
ABG	Arterial PO_2 low

CHRONIC PULMONARY VENOUS CONGESTION

FEV_1/FVC	Normal
TLC	Reduced
RV	Increased up to 40%
TL_{CO}	Reduced
ABG	Arterial PO_2 low

BIBLIOGRAPHY

Gibson, G. 1996: *Clinical tests of respiratory function*, 2nd edn. London: Chapman & Hall.

A useful text which gives an excellent account of abnormalities found by disease.

Hughes, J. and Pride, N. 1999: *Lung function tests: Physiological principles and clinical applications*. London: WB Saunders.

The gold standard text in lung function testing. Extremely detailed.

Lumb, A. B. 2000: *Nunn's applied respiratory physiology*, 5th edn. Oxford: Butterworth-Heinemann.

The gold standard text in respiratory physiology.

Wasserman, K., Hansen, J. E., Sue, D. Y., Whipp, B. J. and Casaburi, R. 1999: *Principles of exercise testing and interpretation*, 3rd edn. Philadelphia: Lippincott Williams & Wilkins.

West, J. B. 1995: *Respiratory physiology*, 4th edn. Baltimore: Williams & Wilkins.

West, J. B. 1998: *Pulmonary pathophysiology*, 5th edn. Baltimore: Lippincott Williams and Wilkins.

INDEX